TABLE OF CONTENTS

ACKNOWLEDGMENT

The authors wish to thank Mrs. Rawnie Obrigewitch for her invaluable editorial assistance and Mrs. Kay Bowen for her excellent assistance in the preparation of this manuscript. Without their efforts, this book would never have come to be.

Enjoying Life

with
Chronic
Obstructive
Pulmonary
Disease

THIRD EDITION

Thomas L. Petty, M.D. • *Louise M. Nett, R.N.*

Copyright 1995 by Laennec Publishing, Inc., 218 Little Falls Road, Cedar Grove, New Jersey. All rights reserved.

Library of Congress Catalog Card Number: 94-74426

ISBN: 1-886128-04 9

PREFACE TO THE FIRST EDITION

Can you enjoy life with emphysema? Certainly. But you will be best equipped to live and enjoy if you understand emphysema and its treatment.

Today, emphysema is almost a household word. Nearly everyone knows someone who has suffered from its disabling consequences. It can progress to the point of invalidism, leaving its victims straining for every breath. It can ruin the health and happiness of both patients and families.

We counter the above with hope. We know what causes emphysema, how to identify it early, and what to do about it. Today, emphysema can be prevented, arrested, or improved, even in advanced stages. Therefore, we are optimistic about what we and others have learned about emphysema and are excited about the future.

We have written extensively about emphysema for doctors, nurses, and patients during the past 30 years. And we are writing again for both patients and health workers because new ways of dealing with emphysema have been developed. The health of nearly everyone with emphysema can be improved, and enjoyment of life can be achieved. We have, therefore, written this book with the objective of restoring pleasure and meaning to life for those with emphysema and for their families.

Denver, Colorado   Thomas L. Petty
                                                  Louise M. Nett

PREFACE TO THE SECOND EDITION

The prevention and control of emphysema have been elusive goals, even though we recognize the major controllable risk factor, smoking. Today, we are beginning to develop effective smoking prevention and cessation strategies. But we already have 30 million or more Americans with various stages of emphysema in this country today and the incidence continues to rise. Effective treatment for emphysema is now established and it can greatly improve the length and quality of life of nearly every emphysema patient.

The enjoyment of life in spite of disease or impairment is a major goal for medicine and society. The first edition of *Enjoying Life With Emphysema* (now entitled *Enjoying Life With Chronic Obstructive Pulmonary Disease (COPD)*, was directed to emphysema patients and their families so that they could understand the lungs, the emphysema process, and the basics of therapy. How to cope and adapt and still enjoy a full life is the message of both editions. Many new advances have occurred since the first edition—thus the second, to bring everyone up to date. Each chapter has been revised where appropriate and a new chapter on Home Care added. We continue to believe that everyone with emphysema can be improved and can enjoy the life that lies ahead.

Denver, Colorado

Thomas L. Petty
Louise M. Nett

PREFACE TO THIS THIRD EDITION

We are delighted to report real progress in our goals of treating chronic obstructive pulmonary disease and bringing comprehensive care to patients with emphysema and related disorders. Because of a new emphasis on smoking prevention and cessation, we look forward to a major reduction in the prevalence of emphysema, though today it remains a major affliction for millions in our society.

The full spectrum of chronic airflow disorders is best termed chronic obstructive pulmonary disease (COPD). COPD encompasses asthmatic bronchitis, chronic bronchitis, emphysema, and combinations of these closely-related disorders. Blending these "labels" is quite common and often leads to confusion. Thus, we will use the broader term COPD in this Third Edition.

The principles and practice of pulmonary rehabilitation are, at last, well established, and it is now the standard of care for patients with symptomatic chronic respiratory disease who want more than ordinary care. These are the people who want to prevent premature morbidity and mortality from COPD. These are the people who want to continue zestful living. Significant advances in our ability to help patients enjoy life have occurred since we wrote the Second Edition. We dedicate this Third Edition to those with an adventurous spirit, to those who look forward to sunrises instead of sunsets. Tomorrow promises a better day for those who learn to enjoy life with COPD!

Denver, Colorado   Thomas L. Petty
                                                Louise M. Nett

CHAPTER ONE

THE MAGNIFICENT LUNGS

Just about all of us are concerned about our health. Quite appropriately, the heart gets a lot of attention in this area; everyone knows that heart attacks are the number one cause of disability and death in this country. The heart is a remarkable pump that delivers blood to every organ of the body. When healthy, it does its job with a great amount of reserve. The popularity of jogging, walking, and other forms of exercise illustrates our new commitment to health through physical fitness.

It is amazing that only a few people have equal reverence for the lungs. After all, the lungs provide oxygen, which is pumped by the heart and carried by the blood throughout our bodies—even to the heart itself!

• Oxygen energizes every cell of the body. It is key to the energy chain that keeps us living.

• A great amount of the oxygen we take in is used to maintain cell and tissue structure.

• Oxygen is required for all organ functions, including heart functions, that are involved in every living activity. Oxygen is critical to the survival of all human beings.

A shortage of oxygen affects every organ of the body.

• The brain has the highest oxygen requirement of all the organs.

• The heart has an immense oxygen requirement compared with the other organs of the body.

• The liver, kidneys, and all other organs require oxygen for their own vital functions. Thus, in states of oxygen deficiency the whole body becomes robbed of vital energy.

Oxygen is involved in the process of metabolism, which converts food into the energy we need to live. A by-product of metabolism is carbon dioxide. The lungs remove carbon dioxide from the blood as it is returned from the tissues. When the lungs cannot exhale enough carbon dioxide, there is a toxic buildup, resulting in "acidosis," an acid poisoning of all the cells of the body. The brain, heart, and other organs are also impaired by carbon dioxide retention.

Understanding the lungs would be quite easy if they simply exchanged oxygen and carbon dioxide. But they do much more:

- The lungs are the only organ in the body that receive the heart's entire blood flow with each heartbeat.

- As blood from the veins flows to the right side of the heart and through the lungs, many of the body's chemicals are either inactivated or activated by the lungs. For example, the lungs activate a hormone that controls blood pressure.

- The lungs, through their normal function, affect our daily moods and emotions.

The lungs are the largest organ in the body. Their total surface area is more than 100 square yards—the size of a tennis court. The delicate gas exchange membrane, or air-blood interface, is 1/50th the thickness of tissue paper.

Millions of tiny capillaries carry red blood cells throughout the body, transporting oxygen in and carbon dioxide out. These red cells also contain mechanisms that defend against cigarette smoke, air pollution, and other noxious materials. Thus, the red cells are not only servants to every organ and tissue, but they are also the defenders against cancer, emphysema, and other lung diseases.

White cells, which defend us against infection, also traverse the lungs. In fact, at any one minute at least 17 billion white blood cells are cruising through our lungs. Billions are stored there, poised and ready to attack bacteria, viruses, and other infectious invaders that we inhale every day.

Nearly all of us know our height, weight, age, family background, and blood type. Virtually everyone has had his or her blood pressure measured from time to time. Regular checkups of skin, breasts, and other organs can warn us well in advance of cancer. Yet rarely do we have a "lung checkup." If the lungs are so critical to our health and happiness, why do we take them for granted?

Actually a "lung checkup" or vital capacity test is quite simple. The test measures the amount of air that can be blown out of fully inflated lungs. Vital capacity is a better predictor of longevity than other tests, including blood pressure, electrocardiograms, or blood tests. This breathing capacity has truly proven to be the capacity for life. But how many people know their own vital capacity? Testing devices are readily available but, unfortunately, are used too infrequently in physicians' offices. Indeed, two simple devices which cost less than $15.00 could be used by all Americans to test their vital capacity in their own homes (Chapter 3).

The Effects of Smoking

You know that cigarettes are dangerous to those who smoke them. But even if you don't use tobacco, you are not safe from the smoke emitted by someone else's cigarette: passive smoke. Passive smoke contains more cancer-producing chemicals than the air in many chemical factories, uranium mines, or asbestos factories. Cigarette smoke is more radioactive than many x-rays!

A huge number of tobacco chemicals invade our body through the lungs unless we insist upon our right to breathe clean air. These chemicals can cause lung cancer, the most common fatal malignancy in both men and women. The carcinogens are also carried to other organs of the body, causing cancer of the bladder, uterus, and pancreas. In fact, it is estimated that 30 to 50% of all cancer is caused by cigarette smoke.

Besides the risk of cancer, smoking doubles your risk of heart attack. And even if you don't contract cancer or die from a heart attack, you are likely to develop chronic obstructive pulmonary disease (COPD), the fourth most common cause of death and the second major cause of disability in our nation.

Our society spends at least $2.5 billion a year for oxygen therapy and many more billions for respirators in intensive care units. Tobacco kills approximately 1,500 Americans each day. But we continue to allow tobacco sellers to advertise their deadly products. It is estimated that 4,000 people have died in Bhopal, India, since the world's greatest industrial disaster in 1984, but we accept 450,000 deaths per year as a matter of "personal preference." Court dockets are full of claims against the asbestos, mining, and chemical industries. However, our billboards, magazines, and newspapers continue to sell heart attack, cancer, and COPD. Why do we continue to promote suffering and death?

What is the answer to this paradox?

- The first step is to recognize the lungs as major health organs. We must identify lung health as the basis for a healthy, happy, long life.

- Second, we must learn about the condition of our own lungs and be able to protect them.

- Third, we must support legislation against smoking in public places and against tobacco advertising of all types, including the endorsement and sponsorship of sporting events.

Finally, we must continue in our research efforts to understand the basic mechanisms of lung injury through smoking. In the interim, before smoking is dramatically reduced in this country, we will continue to develop and evaluate new methods of care for COPD sufferers, as we have during the past 35 years.

Anatomy of the Lungs

The lungs should be considered "the environmental organs." They are unique in their size and formation, and they interface with all the materials you inhale from the community environment, the work environment, and the personal environment. The lungs are made up of a series of branching tubes that provide the pathways for air entry and exit. These pathways, called bronchi, are exquisite in their design, with each tube branching twice: The major airway or windpipe (trachea) divides into two main bronchi, which in turn beget smaller and smaller orders of bronchi until some 22 divisions result in the final conducting passageways (Figure 1).

The respiratory or gas exchange function of the lungs begins in tiny sacs or folded structures (alveoli) attached to these tiny passageways. These smallest passageways

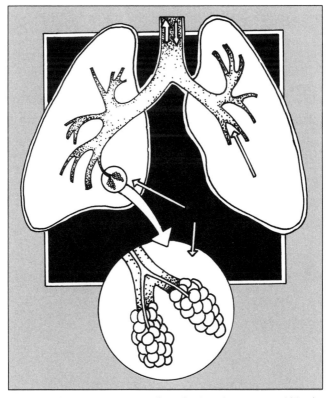

Figure 1. The Lungs: Drawing of conducting air passages within the lungs shows movement of air in and out (arrows) and the small branching air passages that serve the gas exchange portion of the lungs (magnification). Tiny sac-like alveolar structures are folded when the lungs empty and unfold and expand slightly during inflation.

continue to branch and finally connect with alveolar ducts, passageways thoroughly lined by alveoli. Each duct ends in a mass of alveoli (Figure 1 [inset] and Figure 2). The alveolar-capillary membrane lines all of the alveoli and works as the blood-air interface. It allows life-giving oxygen into the blood and extracts the waste gas, carbon dioxide, from the blood. As stated earlier, this delicate membrane is only 1/50th the thickness of tissue paper, thin enough to transport oxygen and carbon dioxide, but still a barrier against fluid formation within the alveolar spaces.

The total surface of the alveolar membrane varies from 100 to 200 square meters, depending on the size of the person. The overall surface area of the alveolar membrane has frequently been equated to that of a tennis court. This

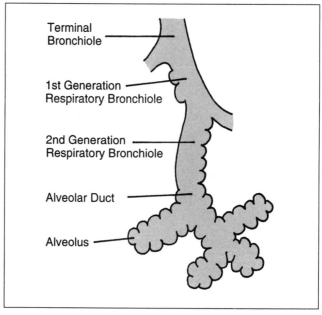

Figure 2. Bronchioles: Schematic drawing of the end of the branching air passages (terminal bronchiole), which end in the first of two or three generations of respiratory bronchioles that begin to contain alveoli. This process ends in the alveolar duct and the alveoli themselves.

comparison is really an underestimation! Thus, the lungs are by far the largest organs that make intimate contact with the environment.

The lungs are also the only organs of the body that receive all the blood from the heart with every heartbeat. Thus, any material in the bloodstream circulates through the lungs constantly. Some materials, such as small blood clots, can injure the membrane and cause the lung to leak fluid. Infections can cause pneumonia, and heart failure can flood the lungs. In these conditions, gas exchange becomes abnormal.

People who truly understand the lungs marvel at their complexity. Consider the roughly 100,000 small air passages that feed a membrane surface greater than the size of a tennis court! This membrane wraps itself around at least 300 *million* alveoli and is lined with a myriad of tiny blood vessels called capillaries. Consider further the fact that approximately four quarts of air pass through the gas-exchange surface each minute, along with some five liters of blood, which traverse the capillary membrane. This magnificent machine occupies the chest cavity and, in all, is some 4 to 6 quarts of total volume. We certainly must consider the lungs the most exquisite packaging job in nature and their function a splendid orchestration. Only the brain possesses greater complexity and capability in design and function.

Naturally, the lungs must be defended against outside damage, and recent research has revealed some fascinating defense mechanisms. The nose acts as a filter, and the conducting air passages contain a protective mucous lining. Within the lungs, tiny hair-like cells called cilia sweep the air entering the lungs almost constantly, acting as janitors. Scavenging cells, called macrophages, are poised and ready to engulf particles that evade the other sentinels. Macrophages are potent obstacles to damage from the environment, but these cells can release enzymes that damage the lung's delicate structure.

Small amounts of normal lung fluids also help the lungs defend themselves. The surfactant system of the lung allows easy filling and emptying of the lungs. Surfactant also provides an antibacterial and immune function to protect against infections.

Within the blood vessels of the lungs, an anti-clotting system combats small accumulations of damaging cells, aggregates, and small clots that enter the lungs from other parts of the body.

Thus, normal lung fluids are being formed and washed away constantly. The lungs have anti-irritants, anti-infectives, anti-enzymes, and immune defense mechanisms, all of which are coordinated to serve these organs well.

The gas-transfer function of the lungs is well-understood today. (In fact, everyone should learn about this process, the essence of normal organ system function. Information on the topic is available in schools and in the numerous health-oriented articles that appear in the print media today.) The biochemical or non-respiratory functions of the lungs are less recognized. We continue to marvel at the hormonal activities of the lungs that, as mentioned earlier in this chapter, regulate other functions of the body, possibly including the brain. Thus, the lungs work in cooperation with the brain, and are the main control system for the body. The lungs are unequaled in their diversity of functions and contributions to the health of the individual.

Thus, the chest, containing both lungs and the heart, is not a "black box." Let's reconsider the orchestration of the lungs mentioned earlier in this chapter. This symphony includes 300 million alveoli and at least 100,000 small airways, as well as the larger airways of the lungs, working together with each breath that leaves our body, some 12 to 20 times a minute. We consider the lungs to be the "pulmonary philharmonic" of our body. The heart, which pumps the blood, is the "cardiac choreographer." For as words flow from a pen and move across the page, so the blood from the lungs is moved by the heart to serve all the organs of the body. But the "pulmonary philharmonic" and the "cardiac choreographer" must have a conductor. The "conductor" is the brain, our most vital control system. The whole human brain, including consciousness and awareness, is the conductor. And, as respiration and circulation are the "recital," metabolism, which fuels all bodily functions, is the "melody." Only the individual can perceive and know his or her own melody, the pitch, the tone, the meter. In illness, we can all feel the decrescendo of despair. Can we once again ascend with a new cadenza and revel in rhapsody? Good music lasts and lingers on!

This brief essay and the suggested reading that follows are intended to stimulate further study, contemplation, and philosophizing about the lungs as the unique organs they are and about the various roles they play in the health and happiness of the whole human being.

Suggested Reading

Scientific:

1. Murray, JF: The Normal Lung (The Basis for Diagnosis and Treatment of Pulmonary Disease). 2nd Edition, Philadelphia, W.B. Saunders, 1986.

CHAPTER TWO

WHAT IS CHRONIC OBSTRUCTIVE PULMONARY DISEASE?

Asthmatic bronchitis, chronic bronchitis, and emphysema are commonly lumped together and called chronic obstructive pulmonary disease (COPD). COPD represents one of the most challenging problems in pulmonary disease today. Lung cancer is the other great challenge. Both diseases are caused by smoking. Tremendous advances promise to change the dismal picture faced by patients with COPD and their families. We can now face all stages of COPD optimistically, realistically, and scientifically.

The purpose of this chapter is twofold:

1. It reviews the current status of our knowledge of COPD as a basis for understanding and for educating patients and their families.

2. It presents a practical approach to patient education. This chapter is intended for patients, for their families, and for professionals, who are challenged to offer comprehensive instruction and care for this important clinical problem.

Background Factors and Causation

The epidemiology of COPD is better understood now than ever before. Basically this is a disease of smoking men and women. Its development covers at least 20 to 30 years in most patients. COPD clusters in families, but the reason for this is not entirely known. Probably, a combination of environmental, socio-economic, and hereditary factors contribute. Environmental factors include smoking, both active and passive, which is—beyond question—the major risk factor. But other socioeconomic considerations, including occupation and general health habits, also play a role.

One hereditary abnormality, called the alpha anti-trypsin (AAT) deficiency state, is now known to be associated with COPD. AAT deficiency often causes disease at an early age. It affects men and women equally. However, AAT deficiency is only one mechanism by which hereditary factors are related to COPD. COPD sometimes, though rarely, occurs in non-smoking families in whom AAT is normal. Thus, there are undoubtedly other hereditary factors that lead to risk of disease.

Information about familial association can be used as a starting point when counseling patients. It may encourage behavioral modification, i.e., smoking cessation, as the basis for preventive therapy, which is particularly important in the early stages of disease to prevent further deterioration of health.

The prevalence of COPD has been estimated to be approximately 38 per 1,000 in the US population. This figure is probably an underestimation. In a survey begun in 1967, we found a greater disease prevalence in Glenwood Springs, Colorado, where 29% of men had chronic cough and expectoration of sufficient duration to justify the diagnosis of chronic bronchitis, and 13% had chronic airflow limitation, a sign of COPD. Airflow obstruction or limitation is the main signal of significant COPD. These studies were drawn from a sample of patients taken at random from the entire city. Women had a disease prevalence approximately 50% of that found in men. However, the prevalence of smoking in women was much less in the mid-60s than it is today. As women smoke more, the risk of COPD rises. Today, the incidence of COPD is rising more rapidly in women than in men.

An exciting development is the advent of synthetic anti-elastases, as well as anti-oxidants. Both elastases and oxidants are believed to be the basic causes of lung injury

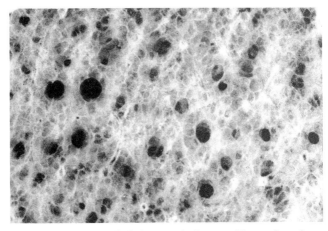

Figure 3. Alveoli: Magnified photograph of a normal human lung shows numerous alveoli around the alveolar ducts. Over 300 million alveoli exist in human lungs.

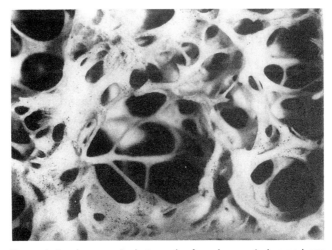

Figure 4. Emphysema: A photograph of emphysema in human lungs magnified to the same degree as Figure 3. Notice the marked loss of lung structure, the holes, the thin remaining strands of tissue, and the dirty pigment contained within the remaining lung substance.

leading to COPD. Synthetic agents will be far less expensive than current therapy. Right now it appears that their delivery by the inhaled route is both safe and practical, although no widespread human trials have yet been done. The future promises additional advances in the field of anti-elastase and anti-oxidant therapy.

Causes of COPD

The pathogenesis (causation) of COPD can best be defined as the destruction of alveolar walls (emphysema) and the inflammation of airways (asthmatic and chronic bronchitis). This is an oversimplification, especially since both an alveolar component and an airway component are present in the majority of patients. Figure 3 shows the normal structure of the human lung as seen through a microscope and magnified 16 times. It looks a lot like a sponge with a delicate structure. The larger spaces are called alveolar ducts, briefly described in Chapter 1. They begin at the ends of the branching conducting air passages, are lined by alveoli, and end in a mass or clump of alveoli, as shown diagrammatically in Figure 2. This is the gas exchange surface for oxygen and carbon dioxide.

Emphysema

Figure 4 shows (at the same magnification as Figure 3) the alveolar structure as affected by severe emphysema. By comparing these two photographs, one can see extensive lung destruction caused by inflammation of the alveolar surface. The inflammation and destruction are the effects of tobacco smoke and other irritants that stimulate inflammatory cells from the blood to enter the lungs and combat the irritation. These cells release enzymes that can damage or destroy the lungs. The enzymes released from inflammatory cells are quite similar to meat tenderizer, and can be used to produce emphysema in experimental animals.

Thus, COPD is a disease that damages and destroys the lung tissue. It affects the surface of your lungs, which is made up of a complicated system of lace-like structures (air sacs) that pass oxygen into your blood and remove carbon dioxide from your blood. In most cases, your lungs can withstand a lot of abuse, and it may take 20 years or more to cause a change in your health.

As the disease gets worse, you have more and more difficulty breathing or you become short of breath. By the time
shortness of breath happens, the disease may be worse than
you think. At first, shortness of breath occurs only with
heavy exercise; later it accompanies light exercise and, still
later, it occurs even with walking or other light activities.

Even if you already have advanced COPD from emphysema,
you need to understand its basic nature. The more advanced
the disease, the less likely your doctor will be able to stop it.
It can, however, still be managed. The chapters that follow
tell how the patient with COPD is evaluated and treated.

Asthmatic and Chronic Bronchitis

Now let us consider the first cousins of emphysema,
asthmatic and chronic bronchitis. Asthmatic and chronic
bronchitis, along with emphysema, are caused and/or aggravated by smoking and, therefore, often occur together.
Asthmatic and chronic bronchitis are due to an inflammation and a swelling of the air passages. These passages become congested and clogged with mucus, and spasm of the
circular airway musculature occurs. Imagine when you've
gotten an insect bite and how it becomes swollen, red, and
painful. Similarly, in asthmatic and chronic bronchitis, the
lining of the air tubes becomes swollen and large amounts
of mucus are produced. Mucus complicates the problem of
chronic bronchitis even more, much like pus in a wound
further infects, clogs, and irritates the wound and delays
healing.

Figure 5 shows a cross section of a small air passage. Its
central passageway is wide open, except for a bit of mucus
in the center. It is able to conduct air in and out of the lungs.
Figure 6 shows a passageway affected by asthmatic and
chronic bronchitis. The air passage is inflamed and plugged.
The smooth muscle surrounding each air passage is also
enlarged. Obviously, moving air through these narrowed
or plugged air passages is difficult, if not impossible. Just
imagine this process occurring in more and more of the tiny
air passages as the disease develops. This inflammation is

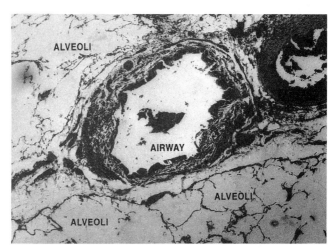

Figure 5. Open Airway: Photograph of an open airway with a small speck of mucus within the air passage and surrounding lung (alveolar) attachments. A small artery accompanies the airway (right upper corner). Small airways and arteries run together for the matching of airflow and blood flow. The surrounding delicate alveoli attached to the small airway are also seen.

the reason for cough, the body's attempt to throw off inflammation and irritation. Bronchospasm, plugged air passages, and loss of elasticity through inflammatory destruction (emphysema) make breathing difficult. You have to work harder to breathe, and as a result, experience shortness of breath. You can now understand why the main symptoms of COPD are cough and shortness of breath.

The muscles that surround each of the tubes often tighten in response to various stimuli, causing bronchospasm. Bronchospasm, like the other problems described, makes the space inside the air tube smaller and decreases the amount of air that can flow in and out of your lungs. All these conditions can usually be relieved or improved with treatment.

The treatment dilates the bronchial tubes by relaxing the circular muscles that are wrapped around the air passages. Drugs that dilate air passages are called bronchodilators. They are discussed in Chapter 5. Avoiding the irritation of cigarette smoke or environmental and industrial air

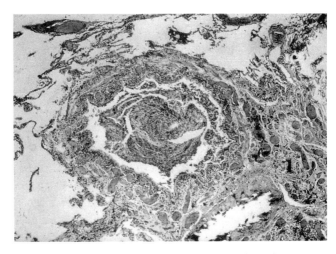

Figure 6. Blocked Airway: Inflamed, thickened, and plugged air passage, which markedly compromises airflow in a patient with bronchitis. Mucus retention is present in this small airway.

pollution also helps. In fact, avoiding the cause and aggravating factors is crucial. Drugs that combat inflammation are in a class called corticosteroids, often simply called "steroids," e.g., prednisone (see Chapter 5).

Educating the Patient and Family

A major purpose of this book is patient education. Thus, careful reading of the entire book can serve as an introduction to, or the basis of further learning about, the disease processes and how to cope with them. This book will stimulate additional questions, however. It will be particularly helpful for you to sit down with your doctor for a few sessions and receive detailed answers to your questions.

Many pulmonary physicians, allergists, and primary care physicians, i.e., internists and family practitioners, have additional reading material for patients and their families. Some offices and clinics are equipped with slide-tape presentations or brief video tapes to help patients and families understand the problem of COPD. But there is nothing quite as helpful as person-to-person interaction with a professional such as a nurse, respiratory therapist, or physician. Patient education requires time and patience, but these are necessary for all learning.

Finally, there is nothing wrong with going to a medical library and reading detailed medical texts. You may not understand *all* the terminology, but you will learn a lot. The glossary at the end of this book will also help. In addition, we have some brief pamphlets for both patients and their families which we will be happy to send to you on request.

Remember, the entire COPD process takes 20 to 30 years to develop fully. Any cough or shortness of breath should be cause for alarm and should send you to your doctor for an evaluation *before* COPD becomes advanced or disabling. You will enjoy knowing where you stand—your lung capacity is the basis of health and happiness in your future.

COPD as a Systemic Disease

Many health care workers with extensive experience in treating COPD have begun to ask the question, "Why not begin to treat patients early in the natural course of COPD, before the late and often irreversible stages of disease overtake the patient? Why not begin comprehensive care, including rehabilitation, at a time when a major impact on disease prognosis is possible?"

In support of the notion that pulmonary rehabilitation techniques should be initiated much earlier in the course of COPD, a recent study shows that even patients with only modest degrees of airflow obstruction have significant exercise limitation. This study presents important new data suggesting that the global impact of airflow obstruction begins early in the natural history of COPD. It is certainly possible that a vicious cycle of mild airflow limitation and resulting reduced activities of daily living create a state of premature morbidity well before advanced stages of airflow obstruction and COPD occur. Couple this with the psychological components of COPD, which include anxiety, depression, and somatic preoccupation, and we have ample evidence to consider COPD a systemic disease.

Smoking, rightfully considered the root cause of COPD, may be used by patients to counter anxiety and depression. Smoking may also decrease food intake, creating a nutritional part to the puzzle of emerging COPD. Reduced caloric intake, protein restriction, and failure to consume appropriate and protective amounts of antioxidant vitamins all lead to insidious, subtle, multiple organ system dysfunction. This dysfunction makes it even more difficult for a human being to cope with an emerging and ultimately life-threatening chronic disease state. Under-nutrition in COPD is associated with reduced immune responses, which lead to an increased number of bacterial and viral chest infections. These infections cause additional metabolic and nutritional stresses on the patient, setting the stage for an inexorable course of progressive functional decline.

To counter this complexity of events, patients with mild degrees of airflow obstruction, as identified by simple office spirometry, can be encouraged and assisted in smoking cessation, exercise reconditioning via simple daily walks, and improved nutrition through smoking cessation and modified dietary intake.

There is evidence that exercise can improve resistance to infection and that pulmonary rehabilitation can mitigate anxiety, depression, and somatic preoccupation, even in states of severe respiratory insufficiency. Improved nutrition can also revive suppressed immunological responses in advanced stages of COPD. Now, a disease that emerged as an avalanche course to disaster can be turned into a detente for patients with early and mild stages of COPD. I have seen several middle-aged people with diminished airflows respond remarkably to a combination of smoking cessation, daily exercise, and an improved diet, high in antioxidant vitamins.

If COPD is a systemic disease, I believe it is time to take a futuristic approach to its treatment. The many interrelated pathways in the pathogenesis of COPD could create a collision course with disaster. Early identification and intervention allow us to develop a treatment strategy aimed at improving survival rates and quality of life.

Suggested Reading

Scientific:

1. Carter R, Nicrota B, Blevins W, Holiday P: Altered exercise gas exchange and cardiac function in patients with mild chronic obstructive pulmonary disease. Chest 1993;103:745–750.

2. Cannon JC: Exercise and resistance to infections. J Appl Physiol 1993;74:973–981.

3. Fishman DB, Petty TL: Physical, symptomatic and psychological improvement in patients receiving comprehensive care for chronic airway obstruction. J Chronic Dis 1971;24:775–778.

4. Fuenzilida CE, Petty TL, Jones ML, Jarrett S, Harbeck RJ, Terry RW, Hambidge KM: The immune response to short-term nutritional intervention in advanced chronic obstructive pulmonary disease. Am Rev Respir Dis 1990; 142:49–56.

5. Petty TL (Editor): Chronic Obstructive Pulmonary Disease. 2nd Edition, New York, Marcel Dekker, 1985.

6. Petty TL (Editor): Chronic respiratory insufficiency. Sem Respir Med 1979;1:1–98.

7. Murray JF: The Normal Lung. (The Basis for Diagnosis and Treatment of Pulmonary Disease). 2nd Edition, Philadelphia, W.B. Saunders, 1986.

Pamphlets for lay persons (available from us on request, Thomas L. Petty, M.D., 1850 High Street, Denver, Colorado 80218)

1. Petty TL and Nett LM: Save Your Breath, America! (Advice for Patients With Chronic Bronchitis or Emphysema and Information for Their Families. 2nd Edition, 1992.

CHAPTER THREE

ASSESSMENT OF THE PATIENT

Here is a personal checklist that will enable you to determine whether you should consult your physician.

1. Does COPD run in my family?
2. Do I smoke?
3. Am I short of breath more than others?
4. Do I cough?
5. When I cough, do I cough up yellow or green mucus?

History

A careful history, with a focus on cough, expectoration, shortness of breath, wheeze, and the duration of these symptoms, is basic. A careful *smoking* history and an occupational history detailing possible dust and/or irritant exposures are also needed. Most patients have had some telltale symptoms for years before they come to a doctor for an evaluation. None of these symptoms is specific or diagnostic by itself. A careful family history in reference to close relatives with COPD is important because COPD runs in families, as discussed in Chapter 2. Some common questions often asked by doctors or nurses to help evaluate the patient are listed in Tables 1 and 2. It is important to talk about the patient's duration of symptoms, lifestyle, work environment, and problems related to the illness.

Physical Examination

A complete physical examination should be performed during your first visit to a doctor. Figure 7 shows one of

Table 1
Questions Your Doctor or Nurse May Ask

How long have you had cough, shortness of breath, or wheeze?

Have you seen many doctors for it?

What are you now doing to treat it?

How many days did you miss from work last year because of the lung problem?

Were you in the hospital for it? How long and how many times last year?

Describe your usual good day.

Do you have more good days than bad days in a week?

What are you able to do when you are feeling your very best?

Who do you live with?

What recreation do you prefer?

Table 2
More Questions Your Doctor or Nurse May Ask

How does the emphysema or chronic bronchitis bother you?

When does it bother you the most?

What have you learned to do that helps you to live with it?

Does it ever embarrass you to have lung trouble?

the authors (TLP) with one of his long-time patients. This patient has participated in a pulmonary rehabilitation program (see Chapter 7) and is receiving oxygen via the transtracheal route (see Chapter 6).

Your physician will thoroughly examine your chest, observe your breathing patterns, and perhaps monitor how hard you are working to breathe (Figure 8). He will note the degree of over-inflation by percussion, tapping over the lungs (Figure

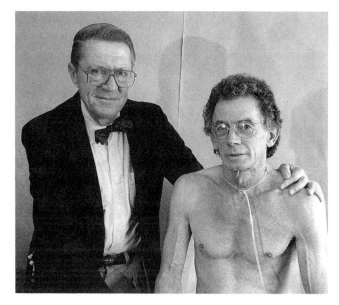

Figure 7. Long-term Patient: Author (TLP) with one of his long-term patients. Notice the use of transtracheal oxygen (Chapter 6).

9). He will listen to your chest with a stethoscope as shown in Figure 10, to hear the air flow in and out of your lungs. The intensity (loudness) of the sounds is helpful. Noises caused by mucus or inflammation are also noted. Figure 11 shows the use of the palm of the hand to note the activity of the heart. Figure 12 demonstrates the use of the stethoscope in listening to the heart sounds to detect murmurs and "extra sounds."

The physician or nurse will also listen to your heart sounds to determine the rate and rhythm of your heart and any signs of heart strain that may accompany advanced stages of COPD.

The examination itself is not very accurate in determining the severity of the abnormality, however. A physical examination may be normal even in the early stages of significant disease. This is because airflow abnormalities are usually moderately advanced before they can be detected with a stethoscope!

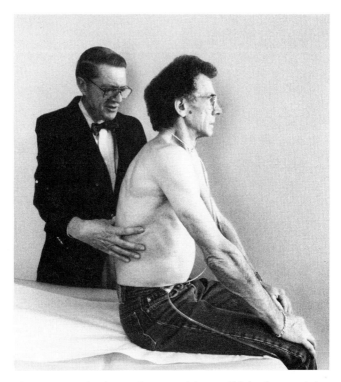

Figure 8. Examination: Patient seated in a well-lighted room during physical examination for COPD. The physician (TLP) has his hands placed on the lower thorax to evaluate the degree of chest expansion.

Chest X-Ray

Chest x-rays are not very useful in assessing the patient with COPD. By the time the x-ray is clearly indicative of the disease, the neighbors usually know the diagnosis! However, the x-ray may show over-inflation of the lungs, which is common in emphysema. X-rays are also valuable in finding other abnormalities, such as shadows, which may indicate coexisting lung cancer. Lung cancer and COPD often occur together because both are caused by smoking. The heart and the large vessels to and from the heart can also be seen on a chest x-ray and give some indication about associated heart strain, but only in advanced stages

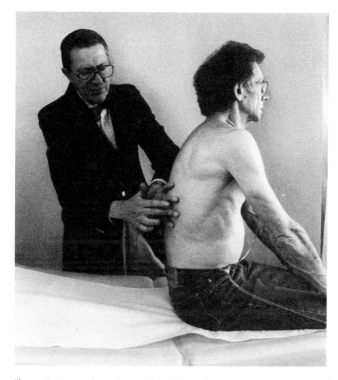

Figure 9. Percussion: The physician is tapping, or percussing, over the chest to hear and feel the hollow sound of air in the chest. This method was discovered by the son of a wine merchant who observed his father tapping on wine kegs to note how full or empty they were.

of disease. However, the chest x-ray can be completely normal, even when the patient has a significant degree of COPD. The x-ray, though traditional, is not a good way of diagnosing or evaluating COPD.

Electrocardiogram (EKG)

The EKG, too, is not useful in evaluating patients with COPD. In very advanced disease, EKG abnormalities are usually evidence of strain in the right side of the heart, i.e., that portion of the pump that propels blood from the tissue back through the lungs to take on oxygen and get rid of carbon dioxide.

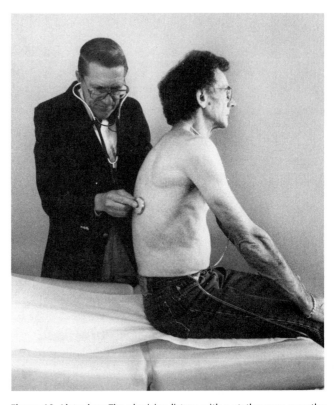

Figure 10. Listening: The physician listens with a stethoscope over the back of the chest for the intensity of the breath sounds and for any unusual noises such as crackles or wheezes.

Sputum Examination

Culturing the sputum of patients with emphysema and/or chronic bronchitis is almost useless. The common bacteria are well known, and today, physicians properly prescribe antibiotics based on their knowledge of the most common organisms and will do so if sputum increases in volume and becomes colored. Yellow or greenish sputum is almost always infected and requires antibiotics. (See Chapter 5 on Medical Management.)

Measuring Lung Capacity

A simple device called a spirometer measures your lung capacity. During this test you take a deep breath, as deep

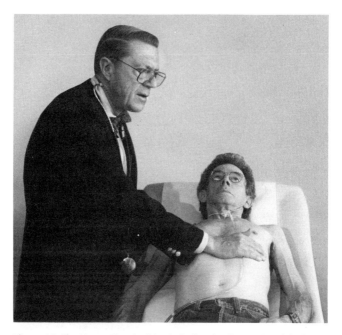

Figure 11. The Heart: The physician is feeling for the activity of the heart. The right ventricle of the heart is anterior (in front) and enlargement or abnormal activity can be noted by feeling each thrust of heart action.

as you can, and blow it out all at once into a machine that records airflow and capacity. (See Figure 13.) Figure 14 shows the actual expiratory curve. Volume is on the vertical axis and time is on the horizontal axis; the flow test (FEV_1) is 2.9 L/sec and the volume (FVC) is 3.5 L. The solid line is the patient's record of airflow and volume. A faint dotted line depicts the normal record of airflow and volume for this patient's age, sex, and height. Note that this patient exhaled for 5½ seconds and the record of airflow is slightly below the norm.

The total amount of air blown out of fully inflated lungs is called the vital capacity. Since the air is forced out by your muscular effort, it is called forced vital capacity (FVC). This test measures the useful size of your lungs.

The rate of airflow tells how open the air passages are and how well the lungs can empty, or how well their elasticity is functioning. The lungs empty somewhat like an inflated balloon. Remember how a flabby or overused

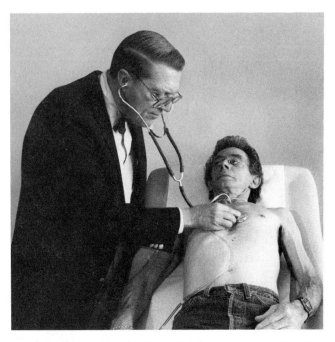

Figure 12. Cardiopulmonary Exam: The physician also uses the stethoscope to listen to the heart's action and for signs of any strain from high blood pressure within the lungs, called pulmonary hypertension. Heart murmurs and other sounds which signify strain on the right ventricle are also noted. The right ventricle contracts to push venous blood through the lungs so that the blood can be arterialized by taking on oxygen and releasing carbon dioxide.

balloon empties slowly and incompletely? This is a lot like the lung with emphysema.

The airflow test is called the forced expiratory volume in one second, since this airflow is timed or measured over the first second of exhalation. The symbol for forced expiratory volume in one second is FEV_1.

These two tests, the FVC and FEV_1, reveal all your doctor needs to know about your lung capacity and airflow. These two numbers are somewhat similar to systolic and diastolic numbers in blood pressure readings. We believe that knowledge of FVC and FEV_1 is as valuable and important to health promotion as knowledge of blood pressure. These tests measure your lung power, which is essential to your continuation and enjoyment of life.

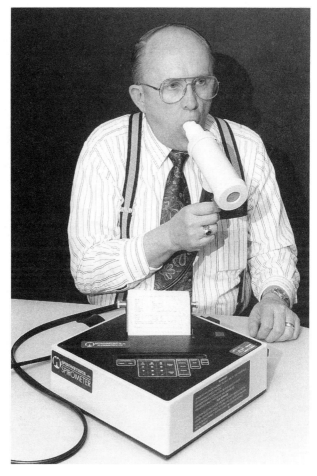

Figure 13. Spirometer: Research Associate demonstrating the use of a popular spirometer. He fills his lungs and blows out forcefully into the flow-sensing device held in his right hand. The record of airflow and volume is traced on the paper; actual values and percentage of predicted normal values are also printed out.

The different patterns of airflow are obvious and are therefore presented to readers of this book to show how simple lung function (capacity) measurements really are. The amount of air, or volume, is shown in the vertical axis and is measured in liters (quarts). The time for airflow (or duration of air expiration) in seconds is measured on the horizontal axis. Flow is amount (volume) over time.

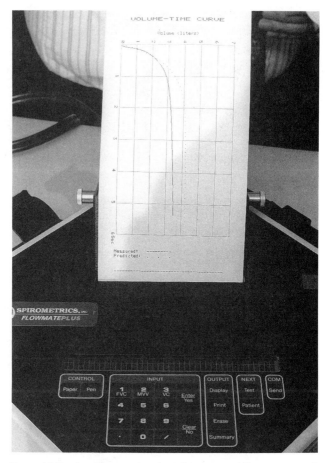

Figure 14. Tracing: The actual tracing of expiratory airflow on paper. The FEV_1 is 2.9 L/sec and the FVC is 3.5 L.

Normal values are based on age, sex, and height. Younger and taller individuals have greater airflow and air volume than shorter or older people. Men have slightly greater airflow and air volume compared with women of the same age and height.

The reader can compare normal lung function (Figure 15) with mild abnormality (Figure 16) and advanced abnormality (Figure 17). The difference between Figures 15 and 16 may take 10 to 20 years to develop, and that between Figures 16 and 17 may take 10 to 20 years *more* to develop. You can see the value of these tests in detecting a deteriorating lung power and predicting the future. If your doctor does not have a simple device for measuring lung capacity, ask him why. These tests are at least as valuable as blood pressure measurements in assessing a patient's health and future.

Many more detailed tests are sometimes used, but they are no substitute for the capacity and airflow tests just described.

Self-Testing – Try It Yourself

Normal lungs have large volume—and they empty quickly because airways are open and lungs are elastic.

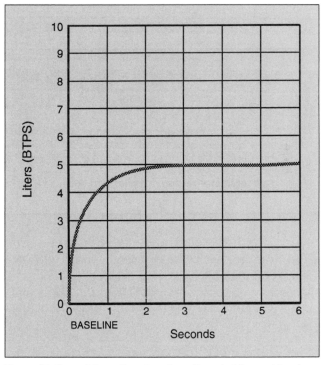

Figure 15. Normal Lung Function: Recording of airflow, with volume on the vertical axis and time on the horizontal axis. Notice that airflow occurs rapidly, with more than 75% of the flow occurring within the first second (FEV$_1$). This is similar to the actual recording in Figure 14. Figures 15, 16, and 17 are from different patients, of course.

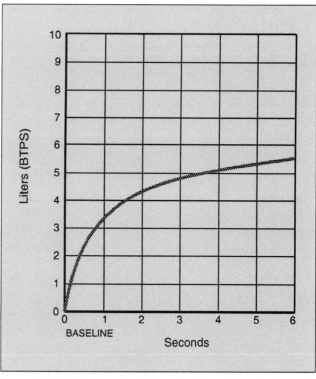

Figure 16. Mild Abnormality: Pattern of airflow with early airway obstruction. Notice that the total volume expressed (greater than 5 liters) is similar to that in Figure 15 in a man of similar size. The first-second airflow (FEV_1), however, is only slightly more than 3 liters (per second), indicating early airflow obstruction.

You can do a little checking yourself with a stop watch. Take a full breath; hold it for a second. Then, with your mouth open, blow out as hard and fast as you can. Your lungs should be completely emptied—meaning that you can blow no more air out even though you try—in no more than 4 to 6 seconds.

If one takes longer to blow out all the air, it means that airflow is obstructed or limited. Today we use the term "limited" because this airflow reduction can be due to either a loss of lung elasticity (emphysema) or problems with airways (asthmatic or chronic bronchitis). See how simple it is!

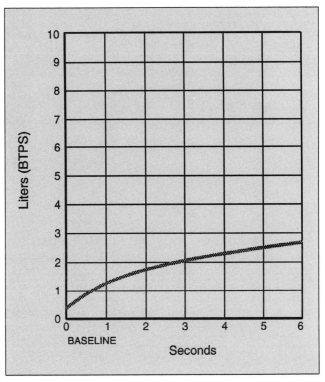

Figure 17. Severe Abnormality: Pattern of airflow in patient with advanced emphysema. Notice that the volume test (FVC) reveals only approximately 2.6 liters and that the FEV_1 (flow test) shows that only slightly more than 1 liter has been expelled in the first second.

Unfortunately, routine lung function tests have been accepted all too slowly. No person would go for a complete check-up if the physician did not examine the eyes, ears, nose, throat, listen to the heart and lungs, feel the abdomen for any abnormal masses, and examine the genital, rectal, and pelvic areas. All these are routine, and to supplement them, appropriate laboratory blood and urine tests are done, plus an electrocardiogram and, usually, a chest x-ray. Unfortunately, none of these examinations or tests identifies early COPD.

Only spirometric measurements of the kind we have just described can identify the patient who is just beginning to develop a lung abnormality.

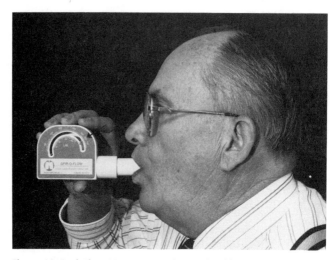

Figure 18. Peak Flow Meter: Research Associate blowing with maximum force into a simple hand held peak flow meter. Note that his peak flow (arrow) is 600 (liters per minute, the convention for peak flow measurements). "Seconds" refers to the key flow test, forced expiratory volume in one second (FEV_1). Peak flow cannot be equated with FEV_1, but it tracks changes in FEV_1 in a given individual.

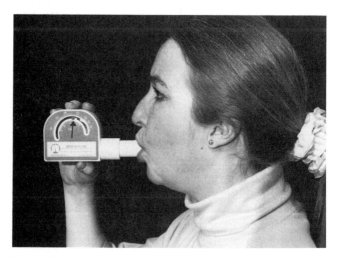

Figure 19. The same peak flow test done by a woman of short stature. Her volume of 370 liters per minute (arrow) is also normal for her.

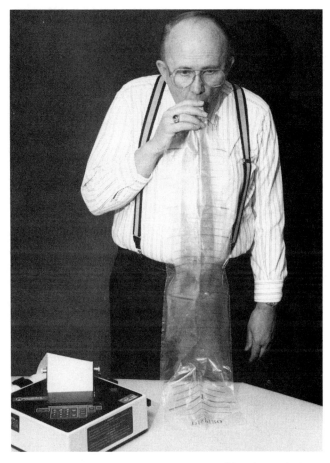

Figure 20. Spir-O-Meter®: Patient preparing to blow into a device to measure the *volume* of air exhaled from fully inflated lungs. This device, called a Spir-O-Meter, is calibrated in liters (roughly equivalent to quarts). The standard spirometer is seen at the left.

When one considers that the disease process finally resulting in disability may go on for 20 to 30 years, doesn't it make sense to identify the problem early and to take immediate corrective action? The answer must be yes if you are to enjoy a long happy life.

Very simple devices for measuring lung capacity are becoming popular. Figures 18 and 19 show one such device,

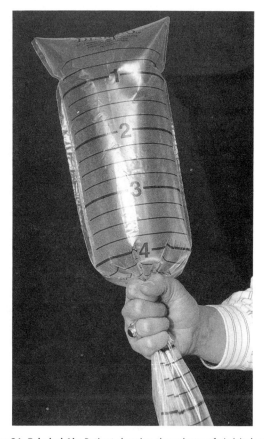

Figure 21. Exhaled Air: Patient showing the volume of air (vital capacity) he exhaled from his fully inflated lungs - approximately 4 liters, which is nearly normal for this patient's gender, age, and height. This is close to the more accurate value of 3.9 L measured by the standard spirometer (Figure 14). Results from this crude device vary from standard spirometer measurements by up to 10%.

called a peak flow meter, which measures the greatest airflow rate you can produce. Note that the man's peak flow is 600 liters per minute (arrow) and the woman's is 370 liters per minute. Both are normal. The lower value for the woman is because of her shorter stature and female sex. Some physicians instruct their patients to use these peak flow meters at home to study their responses to treatments designed to open up the air passages (see Chapter 5 on Medical Management). Another new device called a Spir-

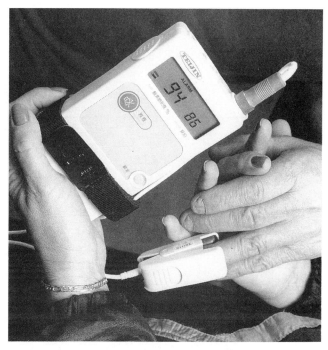

Figure 22. Pulse Oximeter: The oximeter uses an ear or finger probe to reflect two wave lengths of light which measure the oxygen saturation of arterial blood. Note the saturation is 94 - under the alarm indicator. (Normal is 92% for Denver, 94–98% for sea level). The pulse rate is 86. Alarm units can be adjusted to cause an audible signal if lower levels of oxygen saturation or pulse rates are noted by the oximeter.

O-Meter accurately measures forced vital capacity (FVC) (Figures 20 and 21). These measurements of both volume capacity (FVC) and flow can give a good estimate of the mechanical function of the lungs.

Other tests are used in more advanced stages of disease to obtain additional knowledge about the lungs' function. One such test is the blood gas measurement. A small amount of blood is drawn from an artery by a small needle and syringe. This blood is analyzed to measure the amount of oxygen and carbon dioxide it contains. This test is used to assess more advanced stages of emphysema and chronic bronchitis and is needed when the physician is considering prescribing oxygen (see Chapter 6), and in cases of serious and emergency illness.

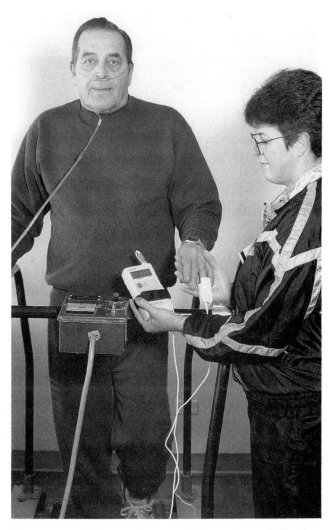

Figure 23. Treadmill: A COPD patient walking on the treadmill with an oximeter monitoring oxygen saturation and pulse rate. This allows for continuous visual monitoring of oxygen saturation (amount) and pulse rate. A respiratory therapist is conducting the exercise test and is holding the oximeter in her left hand and the patient's hand with the finger probe attached in her right hand.

Another simple method of measuring blood oxygen is with an instrument called an oximeter, which is widely used today (Figures 22 and 23). It is popular because it does not require arterial blood sampling. However, it is not as accurate as arterial blood measurements and it tells nothing about the levels of carbon dioxide or acid (pH) in the blood.

The pulse oximeter measures blood oxygen by reflected light. This test is easy and painless and will be much more widely used in the future.

Additional lung function tests such as the *diffusion* test also measure the integrity of the air-blood interface, or alveolar-capillary membrane. Numerous additional tests are used for research purposes, but they do not have any practical value at the present time.

In summary, adequate evaluation of patients with all stages of COPD is within the reach of all doctors and their patients. The approach is simple and straightforward. All patients with shortness of breath, cough, wheeze—particularly those with a family history of COPD and *absolutely* all smokers—should insist on this crucial evaluation.

Suggested Reading

Scientific:

1. Hodgkin JE & Petty TL (eds): Chronic Obstructive Pulmonary Disease: Current Concepts. Philadelphia, W.B. Saunders, 1987.

Non-Scientific:

1. Buist AS, Petty TL, Widemann HP: COPD: Don't wait until it's obvious. Patient Care 1991;25:60–85.

CHAPTER FOUR

SMOKING CESSATION

Americans are smoking less! That's the good news! Nevertheless, approximately 48 million Americans continue to smoke and approximately 3,000 more teenagers start every day. Approximately 1,500 smokers die each day. Millions suffer. That's the bad news.

Many patients with disease do quit smoking, but some think it is too late for them to quit. The fact is that almost everyone benefits from quitting, at any age—at any time. Patients with emphysema and chronic bronchitis usually are finally successful in quitting. However, approximately 15 to 25% of such patients continue to smoke! Many feel guilty and ashamed but continue to smoke, usually because they are addicted. They try to quit, but cannot do so using willpower alone. Some go to stop-smoking classes, looking for help. Some turn to their physician for support. Many have tried nicotine gum or nicotine patches. A few have visited hypnotists or turned to acupuncture. Others have tried a staple in the ear or herbal teas. We often hear, "I've done everything I can to quit." This leads to a defeatist attitude and feeling of hopelessness.

Stopping smoking is not a single event, but rather a complex process. When we do a careful history with a smoker who has tried to quit many times, we often uncover a problem. The history of the quit attempt and a history of why the person relapsed—went back to smoking—give clues to helping on the next attempt. We hear that a smoker decided to quit and decided to tough it out; then only lasted two days. Or the person picked a quitting date during the most stressful work week of the year. We hear sad stories of physical misery endured while trying to quit smoking.

Smokers can use these stories to develop a plan for their next quit effort.

It is useful for the smoker to know some things about tobacco, nicotine, and cigarettes. Perhaps the biggest misunderstanding about smoking is related to so-called low nicotine cigarettes. Most such brands actually contain a lot of nicotine. They can be registered as low nicotine because they are tested in a smoking machine that draws very small breaths at regular intervals. Also, these cigarettes are made from porous paper with minute holes around the filter.

Humans smoke differently than machines. They take deeper breaths, burn the ash hotter, and volatilize more nicotine. Smokers often hold the cigarettes in their fingers while inhaling. The fingers cover the pin holes around the filter, so the smoke is not diluted with room air.

Researchers have measured nicotine levels in the blood of low nicotine and high nicotine cigarette smokers and have not found a difference. Why? Perhaps because many smokers who switch to low nicotine cigarettes increase their cigarette consumption. So, instead of smoking a pack of 20 cigarettes, they smoke 28–30 cigarettes, or even two packs, a day. This increase elevates not only their level of nicotine, but also their intake of carbon monoxide and other toxins.

Carbon Monoxide

Carbon monoxide is an odorless, poisonous gas formed when substances are burned. It is emitted from car mufflers, and is the main reason for opening your garage door before starting your car. In polluted cities, we are concerned when the level of carbon monoxide in the air we breathe reaches 15 or 16 parts per million. Yet some pack-a-day smokers constantly achieve levels of 24 to 35 parts per million! This number increases dramatically right after a cigarette is smoked, often to 80 or 100 parts per million!

The carbon monoxide gas molecule is more easily picked up by red blood cells than is oxygen. So patients with lung disease who continue to smoke have lower levels of circulatory oxygen. One study from Great Britain showed that COPD patients who continued to smoke while receiving oxygen therapy did not reap all of its benefits. Their higher levels of hemoglobin or polycythemia showed up as thicker blood, which puts a strain on the heart.

Patients on oxygen should never smoke because of the possible fire hazard. We recall one woman who was slightly confused and lit her nasal oxygen cannulae instead of her cigarette. She received a rather serious facial burn.

Why People Smoke

People start to smoke and continue to smoke for a variety of reasons. Most children experiment with cigarettes. Some find their first experience a nauseating event and want nothing more to do with cigarettes. Some are nauseated, but get a buzz or high and continue to try to learn to smoke. After smoking as few as 100 cigarettes some teenagers are hooked, and smoking becomes a life-long habit for most. Teenagers and young adults rarely try to quit smoking. Young people think cigarettes help them concentrate, but recent research shows that is not true. Some people use cigarettes to manage weight—an unhealthy thing to do!

Some smokers say cigarettes give them pleasure. It is their only bad habit. They like cigarettes! Nicotine does modify the mood of chronic users. In fact, we are now concerned that many smokers experience depression when they stop smoking. Depression has long been associated with COPD, and some researchers theorize that it is masked by smoking and reveals itself upon cessation. Anyone with a history of depression should seek medical and/or psychiatric advice when making an attempt to quit smoking. Antidepressants, along with nicotine replacement, may help.

Levels of Smokers

We tend to lump all smokers into one category, i.e., a person is either a smoker or a non-smoker. However, there are different levels of smokers. There are light smokers, who smoke about 15 cigarettes a day. They have the easiest time quitting smoking. *Heavy* smokers use more than a pack of cigarettes a day. They have the hardest time quitting.

One might categorize the light smoker as less dependent. Usually, the less dependent smoker can wait 30 minutes before having a cigarette after awakening, has no trouble with smoking restrictions, can go for hours between cigarettes, and does not experience physical discomfort when abstinent from cigarettes. The dependent smoker needs high doses of nicotine and more cigarettes, smokes within a few minutes of arising, smokes every couple of hours, avoids places where smoking is restricted, smokes every day, and feels miserable (suffers withdrawal symptoms) when not allowed to smoke for three or four hours. The dependent smoker is chemically dependent on nicotine. This smoker may need nicotine replacement, such as Nicorette® or nicotine patches, at quitting time.

There is another type of smoker that puzzles the research community—the chipper. This type of smoker can go for days without a cigarette, then can have a few puffs or a pack of cigarettes. This smoker does not get a "high" from smoking, and does not experience withdrawal symptoms when not smoking. This smoker can take or leave cigarettes. We wonder why the chipper bothers to use cigarettes. What do they do for him or her? Most chemically dependent smokers, those who need the nicotine, want to be chippers. However, dependent smokers cannot limit themselves to an occasional cigarette.

Addiction

When the brain's nicotine receptors receive the message that nicotine is in the bloodstream, they are very demanding of the chemically dependent smoker. A little bit of nicotine is not satisfying. These nicotine receptors want more and more nicotine. When the nicotine dependent smoker quits, it must be forever. Teasing these receptors with occasional puffs is a crazy thing to do.

Nicotine is a strongly addicting substance. Canada was the first country to label cigarette packages with this warning. The Surgeon General's report in 1988 reviewed all the medical literature about nicotine's addicting characteristics. The main points of this large volume of work are:

1. Nicotine dependent smokers use tobacco (cigarettes) every day.

2. The drug nicotine can cause changes in mood.

3. Dependent smokers will use tobacco even when they have a disease made worse by smoking, i.e., emphysema, diabetes, or cardiac problems. Actually, most addicted smokers know they are dependent. They want to know how to quit.

4. The craving for cigarettes may persist after a person stops smoking.

5. Relapse (going back to smoking) is common in dependent smokers.

Quitting smoking is a process that happens over time. The decision to quit is based on personal reasons and public pressure. The health reasons to quit for anyone with a disease should be enough to convince them, but often they are not. Sometimes learning about the benefits of quitting is more helpful. For example, COPD patients who are taking theophylline should have their blood level measured a day or two after quitting. It is surprising how fast they will be able to reduce their intake of theophylline to maintain an adequate blood level. Nicotine increases the body's metabolism and stimulates certain enzyme systems in the liver. Thus, smokers metabolize theophylline more rapidly than non-smokers.

Passive Smoking

We now know the risks of passive smoking. Second-hand smoke, or environmental tobacco smoke (ETS), has finally been declared a cancer-causing agent by the Environmental Protection Agency (EPA). Non-smoking spouses of smokers are especially vulnerable to heart attack deaths, lung cancer deaths, and exacerbations of asthma. Children of smoking parents have more upper respiratory tract infections, have stunted lung growth and, if asthmatic, are admitted to the hospital more often than children of non-smokers. In many homes, grandparents are forced to smoke outside when visiting their health-conscious children and grand-children. This can be strong motivation to quit.

Motivation to quit and visualizing success are strongly tied to becoming an ex-smoker. It is a good idea to write down your reasons for quitting on paper and place them on the bulletin board or refrigerator. Add to this list over a couple of weeks; you'll probably come up with a long list. Smokers on a fixed income may be motivated by the cost of cigarettes and tobacco paraphernalia, burn holes in clothing and furniture, and the increased costs of automobile, home and life insurance. This is no small matter, as cigarette prices are bound to increase to cover the public health costs of smokers.

Self-Help Books

The "planning to quit" stage is a good time to gather information on how to quit successfully. There are many excellent self-help books available for free or at modest cost. *Clear Horizons* is a self-help book developed specifically for people older than 50 years of age. It is available from your local American Lung Association or the Office on Smoking and Health in Atlanta, Georgia. This 50-page booklet is packed with good advice.

The National Cancer Institute has a smaller book designed for all smokers, called *Clearing the Air*, and a self-test, *Why Do You Smoke?* These are free; just call 1–800–4-CANCER.

Your local bookstore or library will also have a large selection of materials. Two of our favorites are Dr. Tom Ferguson's the *No Nag, No Guilt Quitting Book* and *Helping Smokers Get Ready To Quit.* Your local chapter of the American Cancer Society, American Heart Association and American Lung Association may also have self-help videos they will lend to you.

Developing your personal action plan for dealing with urges to smoke, desires to smoke, boredom, and sadness is key to making the process of quitting successful. Think of things you can do to distract yourself. Any hand activity can be helpful. Diversions such as tying flies for yourself or fishermen friends, quilting, knitting, crocheting, painting, and playing cards are good. Getting away from urges to smoke, like moving to another chair or room, can help. Probably the best strategy is taking deep breaths, which stretch the lungs' muscles and nerves just like inhaling deeply on a cigarette.

We all use self-talk to talk ourselves into doing work that must be done, to calm ourselves when frightened, or to handle any difficult situation. It is essential that smokers start practicing this useful coping tool. It is good to *practice* coping skills before you quit.

To reduce your consumption of cigarettes, begin to self-impose restrictions on where you smoke:

No smoking around grandchildren or any other children.

Delay smoking on awakening. Observe no smoking in bed rules. (No one should ever smoke in bed. Most burn deaths are caused by a cigarette smoker who falls asleep with a lit cigarette.)

Never smoke while driving a car. Recent research shows that even young smokers' reaction time is delayed after smoking. Smoking does not improve your ability to drive; it hinders it. Adults' reaction time decreases with age, and smoking further impairs it. Do not become a driving fatality because of smoking.

Once you have learned to control smoking in certain places and at certain times, you will gain confidence in your ability to become the master of your smoking addiction.

Nicotine Replacement Therapy

Nicotine replacement therapy has been available since the mid 1980s. Nicotine in a gum-base, polacrilex, is sold as Nicorette®. Nicotine transdermal systems, better known as patches, came on the market in the early 1990s. Millions have used these aids to quitting. Nicotine replacement helps ease withdrawal symptoms so that the smoker doesn't suffer the physical discomfort of quitting. Since he or she is able to quit in comfort, he or she can concentrate on unlearning a bad habit. Old habits are more easily broken if replaced with new ones, preferably healthy new ones. Try some of the coping techniques suggested earlier.

The withdrawal symptoms of nicotine abstinence include craving, irritability, frustration, anger, anxiety, difficulty concentrating, and increase in appetite. If these symptoms are not relieved, it is because the nicotine replacement dosage is not strong enough to maintain the nicotine levels in the blood to which the smoker is accustomed. It is a good idea for all smokers to gradually decrease their cigarette usage to less than one pack per day before finally quitting. Heavy smokers may have to cut back slowly over a couple of weeks. Most dependent smokers will experience withdrawal if they try to wean themselves too quickly or if they smoke fewer than 12 cigarettes per day. Replacement therapy can start once intake is cut to 15 cigarettes, but do not smoke while using nicotine replacement, especially the patch.

Nicotine in the gum, Nicorette, can only be absorbed in the mouth. Chewing it immediately after eating or drinking should be avoided because food and drink create an acidic environment in the mouth, which blocks the absorption of nicotine. It takes 20 to 30 minutes of slow chewing to release nicotine from the gum base, so it is best to use the gum before you start to experience symptoms. Start with a piece first thing in the morning, then chew additional pieces approximately every hour or two during the day. Many people need more in the morning than later in the day.

The main problem with nicotine gum seems to be under-dosing. Smokers were not afraid to use 20 to 40 cigarettes a day, but are afraid to use 10 to 20 pieces of gum. This seems strange to us, since the 2 mg of nicotine in a regular dosage of gum is not completely absorbed in one hour's chewing. Smokers achieve only one third the blood level of nicotine from gum that they would from cigarettes. The new 4 mg dosage gum can achieve approximately two-thirds the blood level of nicotine achieved through smoking.

The nicotine skin patch has some special advantages and some drawbacks. The main value of the patch is that it provides a constant blood level of nicotine. Sometimes

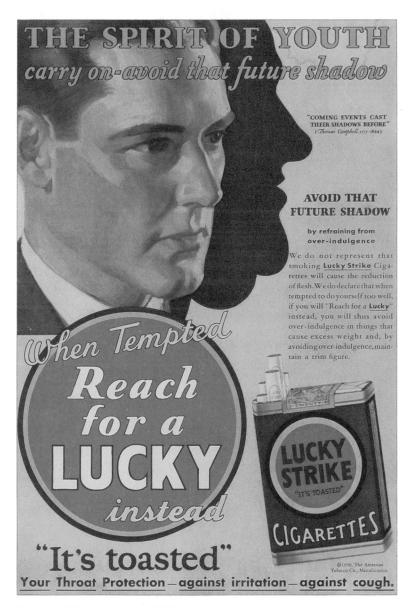

Figure 24. Old Lucky Strike ad (1930).

HAVE A 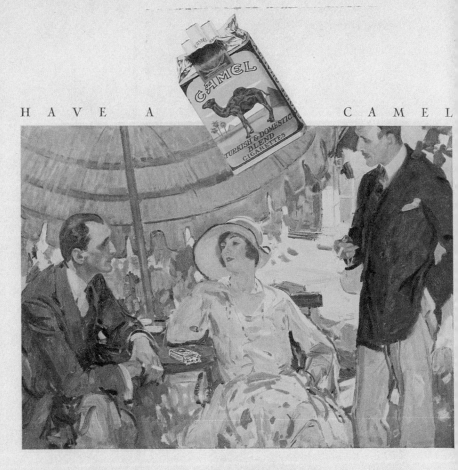 CAMEL

"*Personally, I smoke for pleasure.*

When enjoyment is the first

consideration, the overwhelming choice is

CAMEL

© 1928, R. J. Reynolds Tobacco
Company, Winston-Salem, N.C.

Figure 25. Old Camel ad (1928).

patients are more compliant with medication when taken only once a day. On the other hand, nicotine gum may be beneficial because of the ritual of using it frequently throughout the day, similar to the smoking ritual.

There are some contraindications to the use of nicotine replacement, so be sure to talk with your doctor or care provider about this. Of course, smoking itself will be even more dangerous once you start replacement therapy. You and your physician must evaluate your treatment options, given your own personal circumstances and health profile.

Other Strategies

Quitting day is a wonderful opportunity for celebration. It is a good idea to line up support from friends and relatives for the occasion. Plan your first day as a non-smoker. Prepare coping strategies and escape strategies to get you out of difficult situations. You're not preordained to give in to your urge to smoke, but without a plan, most smokers do relapse.

Humor therapy is a wonderful tool for everyone. Plan to enjoy at least 10 new belly laughs during the first two weeks after you quit. Rent silly videos or buy inexpensive ones, and start your day with five minutes of Daffy Duck or your favorite humorist. Call up an old friend who always makes you laugh, even if you have to splurge on a long distance call. Laughter, like smoking, releases endorphins, a brain chemical that makes us feel better. You need these endorphins for a successful quit effort.

If you have a pet, get ready for quit day by giving Fifi or Fido a bath. Keep your pet close and handle him or her a lot; it will help calm you. If you don't have a pet, cuddle a soft, squeezable stuffed animal like a teddy bear. If you were lonely during your last quit effort, you know this can help.

Prayer and a belief in a higher power are particularly helpful to some people. Private or public prayer can elevate the process of quitting to a spiritual level. We have heard from many people that it was the key to their success.

Smokers should love themselves for making the effort to quit and should forgive themselves if they slip. One puff on a cigarette can be the first step to a full blown relapse, but it doesn't have to be. It is only when the slip causes you to say "Oh, what the heck—I knew I couldn't do it" that you will slide back into smoking. Those who say, "I shouldn't have had a puff and I'm not going to finish this cigarette" can keep on track. Of course, it is best never to have a puff and stimulate the nicotine receptors. As we said, using coping skills and an action plan can help.

Unfortunately, the tobacco industry continues its relentless campaign to induce young, healthy people into an addicting and life-threatening habit. The ads of the past clearly set the stage for the seduction of our youth into the misconception that smoking is healthy and sexy (Figures 24 and 25). This strategy entices 3,000 teenage smokers each day, even though many of the models featured in Marlboro ads have died of lung cancer, COPD, and heart attack!

Smokers are most vulnerable to relapse during the first week of cessation, with the risk gradually decreasing over the next couple of weeks. Twenty-five to thirty percent of smokers will finally succeed in quitting. The interesting thing is that for each quit effort, the success increases. Most smokers will have to try three or four times in order to stay off for one year. At one year, we can give smokers the good news that, statistically, they have a good chance of staying cigarette-free for good.

Suggested Reading

Scientific:

1. Petty TL: It's Never Too Late to Stop Smoking; But How Old Are Your Lungs? JAMA 1993;269:2785.

2. Kenford SL, Fiore MC, Joranby DE, et al: Predicting Smoking Cessation: Who Will Quit With and Without the Nicotine Patch. JAMA 1994;271:589–594.

3. Pierce JP, Lee L, Gilpin EA: Smoking Initiation By Adolescent Girls: 1944–1988. JAMA 1994;271:608–611.

4. Hurt RD, Dale LC, Frederickson MD, et al: Nicotine Patch Therapy for Smoking Cessation Combined With Physician Advice and Nurse Follow-Up. JAMA 1994; 271: 595–600.

CHAPTER FIVE

MEDICAL MANAGEMENT

Perhaps nowhere in patient care is a practical and systematic approach to management more important than in the case of COPD. We have been intimately involved in the COPD problem for more than 35 years, and the discussion that follows is based on this experience. The stages of treatment are based on our own studies and on our pioneering rehabilitation program, which began in 1966 in Denver. We have drawn heavily on these experiences for the details of treatment presented in this chapter.

It should be perfectly clear from the description of the basic nature of COPD discussed in Chapter 2 that this compelling and possibly life-threatening disease heavily impacts the patient and his or her family. Therefore, a comprehensive approach to treatment is required. The need for an adventurous and thoughtful approach to both patient and family education forms the basis of comprehensive care. Emphasis is placed on the various steps in care, but all facets of medical management are interrelated.

Patient and Family Education

By far the most important aspects of good medical care for COPD are detailed instructions and general health education for the patient and his or her family. The basic nature of the disease, the goals of therapy, and the details of management must be outlined in an understandable way. This is one of the main reasons we have written this book. Above and beyond understanding the disease, however, counseling is required to outline and explain some of the psychological components of COPD and to encourage and enable the patient to participate in self care. We feel that each patient must become an expert in COPD care. You should be the most valuable member of your own health care team!

Most fundamental of all is stopping smoking, hopefully in early stages of disease. The concept of "lung age" is now established as a major indicator of premature morbidity and mortality from COPD. A personal "lung age" is that chronological age at which a patient's measured lung function is normal. The difference between the patient's true age and the estimated "lung age" is a potent predictor of problems in the future as COPD progresses. One way to portray this concept is illustrated in Figure 26. Stopping smoking now can help slow premature aging of the lung.

Alpha Anti-Trypsin Replacement

The alpha anti-trypsin (AAT) deficiency state, a consequence of a hereditary gene defect, is not a common cause of emphysema. It represents no more than 5% of those patients with severe disease. The advent of replacement therapy, however, offers a new approach to AAT deficiency treatment. The exciting thing about AAT replacement therapy is that it potentially corrects a basic defect, very much like insulin therapy replaces the deficiency in diabetes.

Although it has been established that replacement therapy (known as Prolastin®) can achieve blood levels believed to be in the protective range, it is cumbersome and expensive. Weekly, twice weekly, or monthly infusions can be given; at present it is believed that weekly infusions are most effective. Costs vary from $20,000 to $40,000 per year for each patient, so obviously this form of therapy is out of reach for the great majority of our citizens. Some comprehensive indemnity health insurance programs pay for Prolastin replacement therapy.

Whether or not replacement therapy will alter the rate of decline of lung function is not known, but a national registry of patients has been established that aims to answer at least part of this question. Whether or not truly controlled comparative trials will ever be completed is questionable.

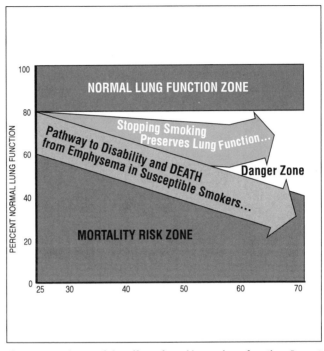

Figure 26. Estimate of the effect of smoking on lung function: Percent of normal lung function is on the vertical axis and age is on the horizontal axis. Normal lung function zone is above 80% of predicted. Any reduction below this level can be considered abnormal. Stopping smoking preserves and may restore lung function. Continuing to smoke in the face of airflow abnormalities has a high risk of leading to emphysema with premature morbidity and mortality. (Reproduced by permission of the American College of Chest Physicians.)

The possible development of an inhaled form of this medication is also exciting, since only 1–2% of the infused material actually reaches the lungs. But we do not yet know whether inhalational administration will be effective.

More on Smoking Cessation

Medications are available to help manage COPD, but stopping smoking is critical. We now have important scientific evidence supporting the value of smoking cessation, particularly in early stages of disease. There have been clear demonstrations that, for patients who stop smoking when they have only mild to moderate abnormalities, the progress of the disease and the rate of deterioration are markedly diminished. Even patients with advanced disease improve when they stop smoking. Figure 26 gives a rough estimate of the increased risk of lung-capacity abnormalities for smokers at all ages. The effect of stopping smoking is also shown for lungs with impaired (reduced) function. When smoking is stopped early in the course of disease, lung function commonly improves and the decline in lung function over time is reduced.

Patients are motivated to stop smoking when they finally realize that something is wrong with *them*! No longer is lung disease a distant intellectual problem, but rather an immediate, personal, emotional consideration. At such time, most patients decide to stop smoking and invest in their health.

The question, of course, is how to stop. Research indicates that the "cold turkey" approach really works best. Tapering off is okay, but you will quickly have to come to grips with the idea of not smoking at all. See Chapter 4 for a full discussion of smoking cessation.

Timing your quit attempt deserves consideration. Most people smoke more in times of stress. Ideally, smoking should be stopped "cold turkey" when things are going relatively well—no deadlines, no great problems in the office, no frustrations. In any case, pick the best possible time for *you*. And begin your "cold turkey stop day" in the morning. Have cigarettes available so you do not panic, but do not open the package and plan not to smoke no matter what.

The first urge to smoke will likely strike in midmorning, following coffee or a meal. *Yet the urge will pass—often in 2–3 minutes.* An excellent diversion is to concentrate on the second hand of your wristwatch for 2 minutes. Stare at it without interruption. After two sweeps, you're likely to find the urge gone, or at least reduced so you can handle it.

Keep using such diversions; use them as often as necessary. It is amazing how the cigarette addiction—and, in fact, it is an addiction—subsides in a matter of a few days for many patients.

Some ex-smokers claim that they never experienced bad withdrawal symptoms, but in most cases the urge gets pretty strong. Simply recognize this fact, grit your teeth, and give the feeling time to pass. Chew gum, suck mints, chew a pencil—but don't smoke!

Also, don't kid yourself that switching to a pipe or cigars will do any good. Cigarette smokers are inhalers. If you switch, you will likely continue to inhale, with the same resulting irritation to your lungs. You simply must decide that all inhaled tobacco is bad for your lungs, bad for your health, and bad for your future.

Also consider that smoking is partly habit-related. We have learned to ask our patients to change their entire daily routine to interrupt unhealthy patterns. For example, if you are used to getting up at 8:00 A.M., having lunch at noon, and dinner at 7:00 P.M., change your routine. Get up earlier or later. Pick a different dinner hour. Have lunch alone if you ordinarily eat with friends. If your evening habits include watching television, read a book instead. If you don't usually go to movies, begin going to them. If you regularly go to movies, change your habit and visit friends, engage in volunteer work, or do almost anything else. The point is to change your daily routine so that you change your habit pattern relative to the urge to smoke. Many executives have found that this works well for them, and in fact, this idea came from a successful executive.

What about passive smoking—breathing other people's smoke? It is now certain that passive smoke can cause lung cancer. Tobacco has finally been designated as a carcinogen by the Environmental Protection Agency (EPA), which equates tobacco smoke to other environmental hazards such as asbestos and benzene. You should sit in the non-smoking area of restaurants and other public establishments. Insist on no smoking in your office. Being in non-smoking environments will also reduce your urge to smoke. Soon the smell of someone else's cigarette smoke will become repugnant, thus enforcing your dedication to saving your health by saving your lungs. It is time that we begin to consider smoking antisocial behavior.

Prevention of Infection

There is considerable evidence that patients with COPD are at high risk of repeated chest infections. In advanced stages of disease, the ability to withstand a serious viral infection, such as influenza ("the flu"), or common bacteria-caused pneumonia is significantly reduced. Thus, infections are best prevented when possible. It makes common sense to avoid persons with colds who are coughing or sneezing. This is not always easily accomplished, however.

Immunization and certain drugs are effective prevention agents for influenza. Influenza-virus vaccines are known to be effective and safe since the immunization effect is not long lasting. Because the viruses that cause influenza are constantly changing, immunizations each fall before epidemics occur are wise. Each year, the pharmaceutical industry produces a vaccine directed against "this year's bug," meaning the predicted strain of influenza. Vaccines have become purer and more potent in recent years. Influenza-virus vaccines are safe, and the complications of the ill-fated swine-flu vaccination program of 1976 have been eliminated.

In addition to vaccines, a drug called Symmetrel (amantadine) is an effective oral drug used against the most common strains of influenza. Thus, if vaccination has not been done or if severe epidemics occur, amantadine can be given during the winter months to protect against influenza.

So far, there are no commercially available vaccinations for the common cold or for other common viruses that plague us all. Considerable research is currently under way, and someday soon we will have better drugs and vaccines against the common viruses that often initiate serious chest infections.

A common bacterial cause of pneumonia can be prevented to a certain degree with a vaccine against some of the common strains of this organism. This vaccine (Pneumovax) is a killed bacterial product and is safe. It needs to be given at least once in a lifetime, and modern concepts suggest that re-vaccination after five years may be wise.

We believe that both the influenza-virus vaccine given each fall and the "pneumonia vaccine" are safe and effective enough that all persons should be considered for these prevention measures at appropriate times. Only known allergies to these products should be considered contraindications. Your own physician should decide about the appropriate use of these agents in each individual case.

Opening Up Your Air Passages With Bronchodilators

Drugs to improve airflow through bronchodilation and/or clearing of secretions are important in patients with all stages of COPD. An important reversible component of airflow limitation is present in almost every patient. Thus, the use of both inhaled and oral bronchodilating agents is appropriate.

Over the years we have evaluated various devices to deliver bronchodilating aerosols. The best method of delivering these agents appears to be a simple device called a metered-dose inhaler (MDI). Bronchodilating aerosols delivered by pressure machines probably offer no advantages and, in fact, present certain disadvantages from the standpoint of cost, complexity, and occasional complications. Pressure breathing machines may cause over-inflation and air trapping and can occasionally cause rupture of the lung. These machines are also easily contaminated and may serve as a source of infection. If there is anything you *don't* need, it's more infection or irritation.

In the distant past, patients were taught to use hand bulb nebulizers, under the theory that they gave a better particle size and avoided overuse of the pressure canister. On the other hand, the relative inconvenience of the hand bulb nebulizer and the likelihood of glass breakage have caused us to turn again to metered-dose inhalers as our standard form of therapy. It is now established that inhaling such drugs as Alupent® (metaproterenol), Brethaire® (terbutaline), Maxair® (pirbuterol), Proventil® or Ventolin® (albuterol), or Tornalate® (bitolterol) is as effective as any other method, and MDIs are extremely convenient to use. Thus all patients must learn to master the use of an MDI.

Table 3 lists the currently available metered-dose preparations by drug and trade names (in parentheses). Table 4 lists the preparations available for use in nebulizers. The techniques of inhaling the medication properly are an important part of patient instruction, which is usually carried out by the nurse or therapist (Figure 27). Certainly, the MDI is the most convenient. Teaching the patient how to inhale this bronchodilating aerosol effectively, however, requires careful instruction.

The patient probably should inhale at a resting lung volume and simultaneously activate the cartridge, continue to inhale slowly, then pause slightly at the end of the inspiration. Finally, he or she should exhale against pursed lips, which helps the deposition of the bronchodilatory aerosol. Inhaled bronchodilators are potent, offer rapid relief, and help to clear retained mucus. They are generally used morning and night, but may be used as well in mid-day and to overcome emergency situations.

Figure 28 demonstrates the closed mouth technique necessary for use of the breath-activated Autohaler® (containing pirbuterol). The Autohaler is more convenient and effective than the open mouth technique for patients with poor press-and-breath coordination.

Recent research indicates that these devices can be used more often than previously taught. If repeated use is required, other medications, such as anti-inflammatory drugs, e.g., prednisone, may also be necessary. A new long-acting beta agonist, salmeterol (Serevent®), has recently been released. Its duration of action is up to 12 hours. Although this new drug may be more convenient than the others listed in Table 3, its true value in the long term management of COPD remains to be determined.

A different type of bronchodilator, ipratropium (Atrovent®), is particularly effective in COPD. Atrovent can be used with the other inhaled bronchodilators listed in Table 3. A combination product containing both albuterol and ipratropium (Combivent®) has just been released. This preparation is more effective than each component used alone.

Table 3

Selected Bronchodilator Aerosols in Common Use
(Metered-Dose Inhalers)

- Nonprescription:
  Epinephrine (Bronkaid, Primatene)

- Prescription:
  Albuterol (Proventil, Ventolin)
  Bitolterol (Tornalate)
  Ipratropium bromide (Atrovent)
  Isoetharine (Bronkometer)
  Metaproterenol (Alupent)
  Pirbuterol (Maxair)
  Salmeterol (Serevent)
  Terbutaline (Brethaire)
  Ipratropium with Albuterol (Combivent)

Table 4

Selected Solutions for Nebulizers

Albuterol (Proventil or Ventolin)
Bitolterol (Tornalate)
Ipratropium Bromide (Atrovent)
Isoetharine (Bronkosol or generic)
Isoproterenol (Isuprel or generic)
Metaproterenol (Alupent, Metaprel)
Racepinephrine (Vaponefrin or generic)

A spacer is not needed if patients use the correct open mouth and press-and-breath techniques or the Autohaler. Spacing devices are expensive and somewhat inconvenient to most patients.

Oral bronchodilators are also used to open air passages. Common preparations are theophylline and aminophylline, available in many brands of tablets and capsules covering a large range of doses. Today, long-acting preparations of theophylline, such as sustained-release tablets or

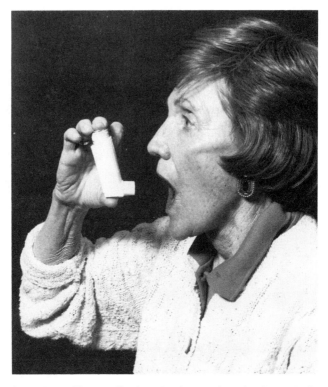

Figure 27. Taking Medication: Respiratory therapist demonstrating proper use of metered dose inhaler. The mouthpiece should be held 3 to 4 inches in front of the open mouth. The patient should inhale from mid-lung volume, i.e., with some air in the lungs, and then continue to inhale slowly. At the end of inhalation, the patient should pause for 10 seconds if possible and blow out through pursed lips.

capsules, are popular (Table 5). They can be used morning and night, and are thus convenient. Oral forms of beta agonists such as albuterol (Proventil and Ventolin), metaproterenol (Alupent), or terbutaline (Brethine or Bricanyl) are also used. They may sometimes help to open additional small air passages not reached by the inhaled product, though this phenomenon is questioned. The oral preparations of metaproterenol and terbutaline often cause more tremor than the inhaled drugs. Tremor, though annoying, is not dangerous and usually subsides in one to two weeks after these drugs are started.

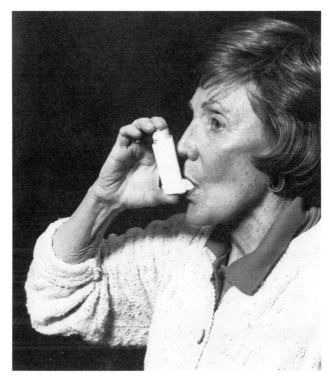

Figure 28. Proper Use: Respiratory therapist demonstrating proper use of the new breath-activated Autohaler®. This requires a closed mouth technique. The device requires activation by raising a small lever between each inhalation.

Antibiotics

The frequent use of broad-spectrum antibiotics is appropriate and should be started at the first sign of a chest infection. Usually, chest infection is signaled by a change in sputum color from white or gray to yellow or green. Usually, cough and expectoration also increase. Routine culturing of the sputum under these circumstances is almost useless. Instead, we have long advised the routine use of antibiotics initiated at home by the patient. Tetracycline, erythromycin, ampicillin, combination products (trimethoprim and sulfamethoxazole—Bactrim® or Septra®), and second-generation cephalosporins, e.g., Ceclor® or Ceftin®, are

Table 5
Common Forms of Oral Time-Released Theophylline

Short-Acting Products (usually taken 3 or 4 times a day)	Long-Acting Products* (usually taken only twice a day)
Aminophylline (generic) Choledyl Theophylline USP	Slo-Bid Theo-Dur Theo-24 Uniphyl

* Many others

highly effective against chronic bronchitis. A one-week trial is suggested. Most experts agree that the duration of infection, as judged by fever and colored sputum, is shortened by the use of antibiotics. These common antibiotics are well tolerated and are not particularly expensive, except for the cephalosporins (Table 6).

Cortisone Derivatives (Prednisone)

In addition to their important role in the treatment of patients with severe asthma, cortisone derivatives, called corticosteroids, are also valuable to selected patients with advanced COPD. The exact mechanism of action of corticosteroids in COPD is unknown, but often bronchodilators work better after the patient has received corticosteroids. Corticosteroids are anti-inflammatory drugs, which may partially explain their effectiveness.

Corticosteroids should not be continued without objective evidence of substantial benefit, meaning at least a 20% improvement in FEV_1 or FVC as measured by spirometry. (See Chapter 3.) These drugs are powerful and weaken the bones and hasten the formation of cataracts. Bone complications, i.e., osteoporosis, are much more common in women than in men. Certain strategies can be used to minimize this problem: Drinking a quart of skim milk each day, or taking calcium supplements like Os-cal® or Tums®. Getting sunshine and exercise also help prevent

Table 6

Common Antimicrobial (Antibiotic) Drugs Used for Flare-ups of Chronic Bronchitis

	Dose	Possible Side Effects
Ampicillin	250 or 500 mg 4 times a day	rash, diarrhea
Erythromycin	250 or 500 mg 2 times a day	stomach upset
Related new macrolides, e.g., Clarithromycin (Biaxin) & Azithromycin (Zithromax)	taken twice or only once a day respectively	few
Tetracycline	250 mg 4 times a day—some other preparations once a day	stomach upset, diarrhea, vaginal yeast infections
Trimethoprim-sulfamethoxazole (Bactrim or Septra)	one capsule twice a day	rare gastrointestinal upset
Second generation cephalosporins-(Ceclor, Ceftin)	500 mg once or twice a day	occasional rash; expensive

bone damage from prednisone. Eye examinations at regular intervals help determine whether cataracts are forming. Glaucoma can also be aggravated by corticosteroids. Regular eye examinations are wise if corticosteroids are used repeatedly or for prolonged periods.

If initial administration indicates that corticosteroids substantially improve airflow, this benefit can often be maintained with small doses, resulting in minimal or at least acceptable side effects. The use of corticosteroids and the development of strategies to prevent or minimize side effects must be prescribed by the physician. Working together, the physician and patient can usually develop a strategy to minimize the side effects of these drugs, maximize their benefits, and enhance the patient's enjoyment of life.

Mucolytics

One recent study has shown that at least one drug that helps clear mucus is effective in some patients with COPD and significant cough and mucus. Iodinated glycerol (Organidin®) has been carefully tested and found effective as an adjunct to the care of patients with a severe mucus problems as a manifestation of COPD. However, the FDA recently took iodinated glycerol off the market for controversial reasons. Organidin has been reformulated to now include guaifenesin, the most widely used and accepted expectorant in this country.

Diuretics

Diuretics are useful if ankle swelling occurs from the use of corticosteroids, which promote salt and water retention in some patients, particularly when large doses are used. The use of Lasix (furosemide) should be tempered, however, because it promotes the excretion of calcium. Older diuretics, such as Hydrodiuril (hydrochlorothiazide), although less potent than Lasix, are effective in most patients with ankle or leg swelling (edema). Hydrodiuril actually helps to conserve calcium. This little-known fact may help to prevent osteoporosis from bone breakdown.

Digitalis

Digitalis is commonly used for heart failure, the inability of the heart to pump with sufficient force. It is also used for some types of rhythm disturbances, such as atrial fibrillation, because it can help to control the heart rate. Digitalis is of little use in cor pulmonale, the most common type of heart failure that accompanies COPD. Literally, cor pulmonale is the heart disease of lung disease. Effective treatment of cor pulmonale must correct the deficit of oxygen, which is the major cause of cor pulmonale. Supplemental oxygen is also helpful in correcting or controlling cor pulmonale (see Chapter 6).

Summary

A combination of patient education, smoking cessation, and drug therapy is now used by doctors to help manage COPD. Medications, of course, mostly treat or prevent complications of COPD. The most effective therapy for earlier stages of COPD is smoking cessation, which will help to prevent progression of disease and thus promote the health and happiness of COPD patients.

Suggested Reading

Scientific:

1. Petty TL: COPD: A new look at diagnosis (Dx) and treatment (Rx) of an old problem. Modern Medicine, 1985 (Feb):128–136.

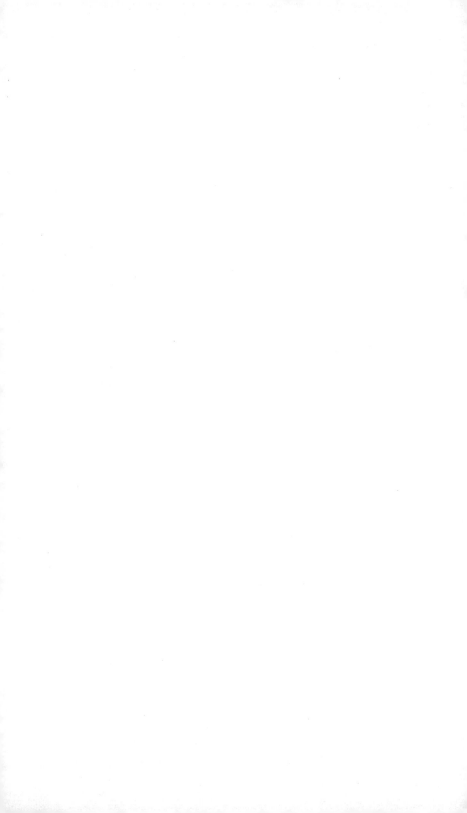

CHAPTER SIX

OXYGEN

Nearly all living things need oxygen to survive, and in fact, we live in a sea of it—the atmosphere. We take nature's oxygen pretty much for granted except when air becomes polluted. Usually we don't pay much attention to the fact that 21% of the air we breathe is oxygen, no matter where we live.

What is oxygen, why do we need it, and what happens if we don't get enough? This chapter is written for patients with emphysema or other forms of COPD who may need oxygen at home, and for their families. It explains the basic principles of oxygen therapy and how additional oxygen in the home can create a new atmosphere for health and happiness.

Oxygen is the most common material in the earth's crust. To a large degree, it is bound to other substances in rocks and minerals. This oxygen is fixed to the earth and is not released into the atmosphere. The oxygen in the atmosphere is made through the process of photosynthesis, which requires a combination of sunlight, plant material (chlorophyll), and carbon dioxide. These ingredients are combined by millions of living plants, including tiny sea plants (algae), during a miraculous natural chemical reaction that releases free oxygen into the air we breathe.

Oxygen in the air is held close to the earth's surface by gravity. Thus, when one goes to higher elevations there is less oxygen, not because there is a lower percentage (always 21%), but because there is less gravity to keep the oxygen molecules packed closely together near the surface of the earth. There is plenty of oxygen, however, for the ordinary person who ascends 10,000 or even 12,000 feet. Indeed, two scenic mountain roads in Colorado climb to over 14,000 feet (Pike's Peak and Mount Evans), and healthy people can be quite comfortable at these altitudes, although shortness of breath, fast heartbeat, and a lightheaded feeling are common with exertion. Sleep disturbances are also common at altitudes above approximately 8000 feet, at least until adjustments, called acclimatization, occur.

Why Do We Need Oxygen?

Oxygen is key to high energy production. The food that we eat is fuel for life's energy. Oxygen is required for these nutrients to be transformed into large amounts of energy. Simple organisms, such as some bacteria, can produce energy without oxygen, but they are inefficient. Since we are complex creatures and maintain a warm body temperature, we require more energy per cell and, thus, more oxygen.

Organized cellular life and its demand for oxygen are sometimes compared to fire. This analogy, however, is overly simplistic, even though fires do require oxygen, produce carbon dioxide, and release energy. There is no burning going on in the body, of course, but energy production (metabolism) does create the heat and energy that are necessary for life. Much of this energy is used to maintain the structure and function of our cells and tissues. Thus, we can consider oxygen a catalyst of life, an essential ingredient of health, and part of our basic energy system. In fact, it is key to our survival.

What Happens If We Don't Have Enough Oxygen?

Fortunately, we have excellent defenses against lack of oxygen. Our first response to a shortage of oxygen is to accelerate our breathing to increase the oxygen supply to the lungs. The heart also beats faster and with more force to carry whatever oxygen is available to the tissues of the body. This is what happens when one travels to high altitude, and this system works well as long as it does not become strained. Long-term exposure to high altitude also stimulates the formation of more red blood cells to carry what oxygen is available, and the essential organs, i.e., brain, heart, lungs, liver, and kidneys, adapt to a low-oxygen environment.

Oxygen deficiency can occur in many disease states. This book and this chapter focus on chronic lung diseases, i.e., emphysema and chronic bronchitis (COPD), where oxygen deficiency is common in advanced stages. These related diseases were discussed in Chapter 2.

Mild to moderate forms of COPD are not associated with any deficit of oxygen, but such deficiency is common in severe COPD. There is no way for a patient or physician to know whether oxygen deficiency is present without taking measurements, although a deep blue color around the lips and nail beds is suggestive. Blood that contains normal amounts of oxygen is usually a deep red, but blood carrying insufficient amounts of oxygen back to the heart is blue.

It is now common to measure oxygen in blood that is removed directly from arteries. This procedure is called arterial blood gas (ABG) determination or, sometimes, just "blood gas." (See Chapter 3.)

The oxygen level in the blood is also measured by its pressure in the blood (also called tension). Normal oxygen tension at sea level is 80 to 90, and at higher elevations such as Denver, it is 60 to 70. The amount of oxygen *carried* in the blood (called oxygen saturation), however, is not directly proportional to this tension because blood can carry oxygen at different tensions. Thus, there is only a slight reduction in oxygen saturation at Denver's higher altitude, where the pressure is 60 to 70, compared with sea level, where it is 80 to 90.

At a pressure of less than 60 the amount of oxygen carried by blood cells becomes significantly lower. At this point, the physician begins to consider whether or not some additional oxygen might be useful. Arterial oxygen is also measured accurately by pulse oximetry, as mentioned in Chapter 3 and Figures 22 and 23.

Other lung diseases, such as the inflammatory and scarring

(fibrotic) diseases, cystic fibrosis, extensive pneumonias, and certain heart diseases, are also characterized by a significant oxygen deficit.

Who Are Candidates For Oxygen Therapy?

This is a key question. By no means do all patients with even advanced COPD require oxygen. Actually, many patients adjust to a small reduction in arterial oxygen quite well. An oxygen level (pressure or tension) of 55 is the usual level at which oxygen might be considered to be useful in patients with COPD.

Even this guideline is an oversimplification. For example, for people living in Leadville, Colorado, at an elevation of 10,000 feet, 55 is normal. This corresponds to an oxygen saturation (amount) of 88%. Remember, however, that most individuals who are comfortable at high altitudes have normal lungs and adequate heart function. Thus heart and blood compensations allow for normal delivery of oxygen to all the tissues of the body. Healthy people can adapt to a significant reduction of oxygen at high altitudes. Physicians generally consider that supplemental oxygen is needed if the level (tension) is really 55 or less or if the saturation is 88% or less after the patient has improved following an infection or some other problem that may have made the individual's condition temporarily worse, thereby resulting in a severe oxygen deficit. It often takes 2 to 3 weeks to discover that the oxygen level is persistently low and the patient requires supplemental oxygen therapy.

Furthermore, we consider oxygen necessary if there is any evidence of strain on the heart as judged by physical examination (see Chapter 3), by an electrocardiogram, or by other signs that a physician can identify. If oxygen is needed, the patient and the family must understand the basic principles of oxygen therapy. The remainder of this chapter is devoted to this message.

How Is Oxygen Given?

Oxygen is generally delivered through normal nose breathing by a set of double plastic tubes called nasal cannulae,

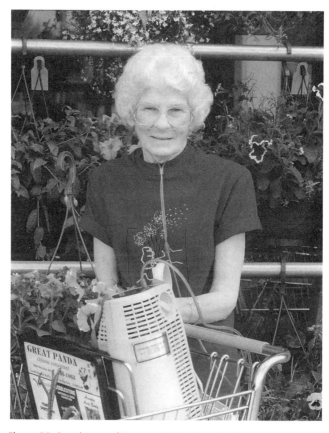

Figure 29. Supplemental Oxygen: Patient shopping in garden store. She is using a double nasal cannulae for oxygen administration. Oxygen is provided via plastic tubing from a portable liquid oxygen device (Puritan Bennett Companion). Some cannulae are used with a small portable compressed gas cylinder (Figure 30) or oxygen concentrator (Figure 31).

as illustrated in Figures 29, 30, 31, 32, and 33. These tubes are positioned just in front of the nose, and breathing takes place in a normal fashion through the nose. It is important to point out that the nose adds moisture and is a filtering system for all air that is breathed. The oxygen that is delivered through the tubes only *supplements* the oxygen from the air. Thus, the amount of additional oxygen needed is small. We think of oxygen *dose* in terms of the flow in liters (roughly equivalent to quarts) per minute. Generally

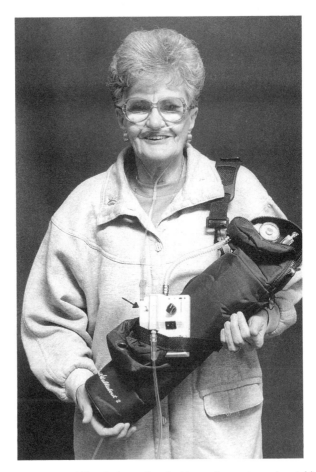

Figure 30. Portability: Patient using double nasal cannulae and portable compressed gas cylinder for "portability". Portable compressed cylinders are often heavier than the newest liquid portable devices and even if used with a conserving device, do not provide as great a supply as do the liquid portable devices.

1 or 2 liters, and occasionally 3 liters, of supplemental oxygen per minute suffice. This is in addition to the 4 to 5 liters of 21% oxygen that you receive through normal breathing. Thus, you can see that this additional oxygen only supplements that which you are normally breathing from the atmosphere.

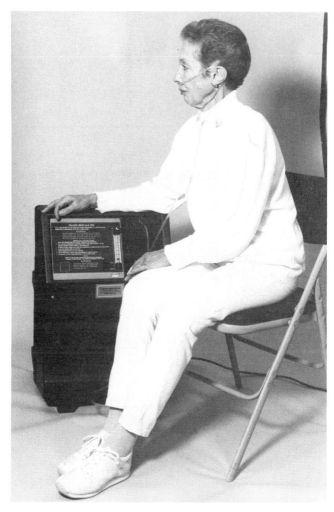

Figure 31. Oxygen Concentrator: Patient seated in a chair breathing from an oxygen concentrator, which produces oxygen from room air.

Getting the Right Dose of Oxygen

Oxygen, like other medicines, must be given in a proper dose. Generally, low flows, such as 1 to 2 liters per minute, are sufficient. Sometimes more oxygen is needed during sleep (when the depth of breathing normally increases), during exercise, or at other times when the demands of

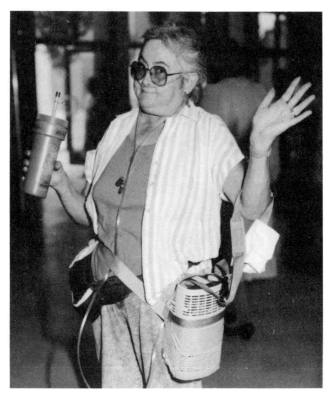

Figure 32. Lightweight portable liquid system (Puritan Bennett) used by a woman at a party.

the body increase. Many experts suggest that an additional liter be used while the patient is exercising or sleeping. This increased dosage was found necessary in carefully performed research studies (see Suggested Readings at the end of this chapter).

The resting dose is calculated by measuring the oxygen in the blood, either by blood gas analysis or by ear oximetry. These two techniques are roughly equivalent in accuracy, but the oximeter does not measure carbon dioxide, the waste gas in the blood. Oximeters are widely used in hospitals that have complete pulmonary function laboratories.

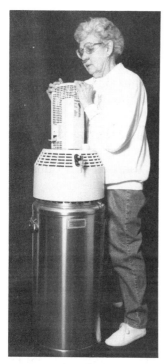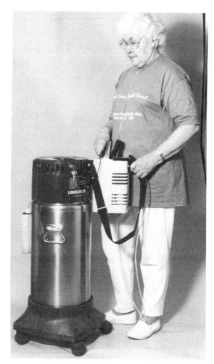

Figures 33 & 34. Refill: Patient is transfilling a portable device from a liquid reservoir using the top fill technique (Figure 33) and the side fill technique (Figure 34). While doing this she is still receiving oxygen from the reservoir device itself.

They are also used by oxygen suppliers as a convenient method of checking the adequacy of the oxygen dose (prescription) in the patient's own home. Now that the cost of oximeters is greatly reduced, many physicians use oximeters in their office or clinic.

• *Getting Too Little Oxygen* – Receiving less than the necessary amount of oxygen is not desirable, of course, but any flow of oxygen, no matter how small, will still add to the oxygen available from the atmosphere. It is often surprising that a low oxygen flow rate, i.e., 1/2 to 1 liter per minute, may actually correct the oxygen deficit. Complete correction of the oxygen deficiency is most desirable. This means an oxygen saturation of at least 90% or an oxygen pressure (tension) of 60.

- *Getting Too Much Oxygen* – Too much oxygen may also be a problem. Some patients feel that if a little is good, more will be better. This attitude is dangerous because too much oxygen can actually reduce breathing rates, leading to a dangerous buildup of carbon dioxide. A buildup of carbon dioxide is potentially toxic, although the body can adjust to slow rises of this gas. Suffice it to say that precision in oxygen dosing is as important as following the proper dose of any other medication. Thus, oxygen should be considered a drug, with the necessary dose to be determined by a physician.

Oxygen Systems

Oxygen is available in a variety of systems, the oldest being gaseous tanks. These are metal cylinders that contain oxygen under high pressure. The commonly used large "H" or "K" cylinder contains approximately 6,900 liters of pressurized oxygen. Thus, one can see that the supply is limited, because in 24 hours the average tank will be exhausted. The need for repeated deliveries also is a nuisance to many patients.

Smaller cylinders are designated by earlier letters of the alphabet. Thus, an "E," a "B," or an "A" cylinder would be smaller than an "H" or a "K" cylinder. A pressure gauge tells how much oxygen is left in the tank. Smaller tanks can be filled from large tanks, and aluminum cylinders weighing only 10 pounds are available. They contain 240 liters of oxygen, allowing approximately 2–3 hours of oxygen supply while away from home (Figure 30). A greater range is possible using an inspiratory control device (Figure 30 – arrow). These conserving devices only allow oxygen to flow during inspiration, so that oxygen flowing during the exhalation phase of respiration is not wasted. Although transfilling of small compressed gas cylinders by patients or family members has been proven safe, any lubricant that might provide material for combustion must be avoided. Unfortunately, the oxygen supply industry and some regulatory agencies frown on this practice.

Liquid Systems

Oxygen is cooled into the liquid form and placed in thermos-bottle-type containers called reservoirs, which are lighter than thick steel cylinders. (All gases can be made liquid or even solid by changing temperatures, e.g., water can be transformed into steam, vapor, and ice.) Liquid oxygen does not need to be stored in high-pressure containers. In the reservoir, it gradually boils and becomes gaseous oxygen, which is consumed by the patient. These systems can also be used to fill portable devices called "companions," "walkers," "strollers," or "liberators" (Figures 29, 33, and 34). The largest of these portable devices weighs 9 pounds and provides approximately 9 hours of oxygen at 2 liters per minute. Higher or lower oxygen dosages (flows) naturally affect the duration of supply.

The liquid reservoir contains a supply for approximately 4 to 5 days, depending on flow rate. Newer, lighter containers, such as the 5½ pound unit, hold less oxygen. Liquid systems are quite popular and convenient. They are the only portable systems that allow for many hours away from the filling source (6 to 12 hours). Liquid oxygen can be conserved by using a pulse control system that is activated when the patient inhales so oxygen only flows during inspiration. The "Pulsair" and Bennett devices are examples of this newer technology. Cost remains a consideration, however.

Oxygen Generators (Concentrators)

Another technology that provides oxygen for patients in the home is the oxygen concentrator. This device takes oxygen out of the air by pumping it through a separating device called a sieve. The process is based on the fact that oxygen molecules are unique in size. The oxygen is then concentrated into a reservoir for use by the patient. The oxygen flows through the liter flow-dosing device via conventional plastic tubing and is delivered to the patient by the same nasal cannulae as shown in Figure 31. Nearly pure oxygen is produced (94% at 2 liters, for example), along with some inert gases (mostly nitrogen and argon), which are also present in the atmosphere. Higher flows of oxygen produce slightly lower concentrations, but the differences are not generally important.

Concentrators are convenient, but they require a reliable electrical source and some regular maintenance. Since they concentrate oxygen continuously from the air, tank and reservoir refills and replacements are eliminated. Concentrators are not very portable, although smaller versions weighing approximately 29 pounds can be taken in the car. Also, 50-foot tubing allows the patient to move quite freely around his home and to get a limited amount of exercise. However, the great advantages of oxygen concentrators are convenience and cost.

Common Concerns About Oxygen Use

The following section lists common concerns expressed by many patients or their families when oxygen is first prescribed.

Will I Become Addicted to Oxygen? The answer to this question is an emphatic no. Addiction, dependency on a foreign material, does not occur. Oxygen is not foreign, and, in fact, it is *demanded* for daily life. We all breathe oxygen from our first day of life. Before birth, oxygen is delivered from the mother's blood supply through the placenta. We must have oxygen to nourish all of the tissues of the body.

In disease states, such as severe emphysema, oxygen deficiency can damage all the organs and cells of the body. Thus, we need to *supplement* the oxygen present in the air using the oxygen systems previously listed. Using oxygen is like wearing glasses to aid in vision. But more importantly, oxygen is bringing to the body the necessary substance for energy. The patient who needs oxygen will not necessarily need it every moment. It is perfectly safe to take the oxygen tubing off for short periods of time, or even longer in early stages of disease. The exact amount of oxygen that should be used each day has not been determined, but in advanced cases of COPD oxygen should be used essentially all the time. Higher and higher doses (flow rates) of oxygen are usually not required by COPD patients. Even in the most advanced stage of COPD, 1 or 2 liters of oxygen per minute are sufficient for the vast majority of patients, with some patients requiring 3 liters.

Will Fires or Explosions Occur? Oxygen does not explode; it only supports combustion. Oxygen, of course, causes an open flame to burn more vigorously, so all flames should be kept away from the oxygen tubing. Patients should not smoke while taking oxygen, and open fires and sparks should be avoided. Unless the oxygen hose itself is directly ignited, however, fires will not occur. Extensive studies of many patients in this country have failed to indicate any serious fire hazards.

Will Oxygen Harm My Lungs or Other Parts of My Body Over Time? The goal of home oxygen therapy is to correct the deficit of oxygen in the blood. Oxygen is given at a flow sufficient to bring the oxygen level near to normal, but not above normal. So far, after nearly 30 years of use in thousands of patients, no evidence of damage to any of the tissues of the body from oxygen therapy has occurred. Thus, oxygen should be considered very safe from the standpoint of its effects on the body.

What About Costs and Who Will Pay? Fortunately, most insurance plans and third-party payers, such as Medicare and Medicaid, provide a large portion of the costs for oxygen therapy—80% in the case of Medicare and Medicaid. Oxygen is recognized as important medicine and as necessary for healthy living. Of course, providing this care outside of the hospital reduces its costs. Although criteria and guidelines for oxygen payment are often under scrutiny and may change, it is not likely that major changes will occur in this country because of the clearly established value of oxygen in the care of thousands of patients.

What Effect Will Oxygen Have on My Life-Style? With a little skill and ingenuity, the use of oxygen may have little effect on your life-style. (See chapters that follow.) Certainly, the use of oxygen should not reduce your activities or hold you back. On the contrary, oxygen should help produce the energy for increased exercise and help expand your horizons. Taking oxygen outside the home is practical and convenient, particularly when portable systems are used. Thousands of patients travel to work on public transportation, drive their own cars, and go on vacations while receiving oxygen. If your doctor feels that you require oxygen all the time, he or she can make provisions for portable systems, i.e., gaseous or liquid, when you are traveling.

Patients can also travel on most major commercial airliners by making advance arrangements with the medical director of the carrier. Oxygen is then provided by the airline at the liter flow prescribed by the doctor. At present, the law says that the *carrier* must provide the oxygen; patients cannot use their own portable system on board the aircraft. However, these devices can be checked as ordinary baggage, picked up at the baggage claim, and refilled at the end of the flight. Fortunately, oxygen suppliers are available in all major cities.

The newer concentrators are small enough to fit in the trunk of a car so you can really "take it with you." In all seriousness, a little ingenuity can allow you to be active in travel, work, and play.

What is the Public's Attitude About Patients Wearing Oxygen? Fortunately, the public has a good attitude about health care in general today. Thousands of people require some form of assistance, including wheelchairs, electric chairs, crutches, artificial arms and legs, and special sight and hearing devices. The use of oxygen in public does not create a spectacle and should not be a concern to anyone requiring this form of assistance to pursue life's pleasures. (See the personal commentary about the use of oxygen by one of our patients at the end of this chapter.)

What if I Encounter Someone Smoking a Cigarette, Someone Using a Cigarette Lighter, or an Open Fireplace When I Am Wearing Oxygen? There is no reason for concern. As stated earlier, oxygen will not explode. It only supports combustion. Oxygen will only allow things to burn if the oxygen tubing is directly ignited. You should be careful to stay at least three feet away from an open flame, but even this precaution is conservative. One could reasonably expect, however, that out of courtesy others would not smoke in the presence of a person who requires oxygen for the treatment of COPD.

What if the Oxygen Tubing Comes Off During Sleep? This accident will often awaken you; simply replace the oxygen tubing. If the oxygen lack is severe, you may awaken with a headache. Since you are still breathing air from the room, there will not be a sudden absence of oxygen for your body. Instead, a gradual reduction occurs as the extra oxygen from your system is used up. It should not be considered disastrous if the oxygen tubing comes off for a short period of time, and even a few hours without oxygen are well tolerated by many patients. Your doctor will give you more specific advice regarding your individual circumstances, but in general, there is no particular danger if oxygen is accidentally discontinued for a short period of time. The same is true regarding electrical failure when oxygen concentrators are used. In areas where electrical failure is common, however, a "back-up" oxygen tank is often kept for these unexpected events.

How Much Good Will Oxygen Do Me? This question, of course, is the bottom line. It is now known that supplemental oxygen provides many benefits to patients with severe oxygen deficiency from COPD. These benefits include a reduction in heart strain, a reduction in excessive blood formation, and improved exercise tolerance. Even the ability to think and solve problems improves with oxygen, because the brain, like all the organs of the body, requires this energy-producing substance. Thus, the benefits of oxygen therapy are many, including improved physical functioning, increased activities of daily living and, most importantly, improved happiness in the pursuit of life.

One Patient's Experience

The following is a prize-winning article written some time ago by one of our patients who lived in Cody, Wyoming.

It explains her feelings about the use of her oxygen tank, which she refers to as "Fatty." These are her own thoughts and words. All people won't feel the same way about oxygen therapy. We have included this personal story because it tells a lot about oxygen as important treatment for one emphysema patient.

"FATTY"

My question is, "Where is everyone?" More specifically, where are the people like myself who are immediately noticed for the plastic cannula they wear in their nose bringing a life-supporting supply of oxygen to their crippled lungs. We are told there are many thousands who cannot function or live without this continued oxygen supply. And yet my husband and I have just returned home from a 6,000-mile trip, driving from our home mountains through the plains and plateaus and river country of the land—and I did not see one other person wearing the familiar plastic hose. (Today you will see many patients with oxygen—approximately 800,000 are using it each day in North America alone.—Editor)

Last winter we made a similar long mid-winter journey and we saw one man coming out of a restaurant at a hot desert lunch stop. He was moving slowly and carrying his precious air tank with obvious care and concern. If I'd been close enough to him, I'd have stopped to greet him—maybe given him a big hug!

At home I get around town to do most of my own errands in our car and I value the feeling of freedom and independence even though I move very slowly indeed. I have yet to meet another person wearing the tube, though I know of several in our small town.

I am coming to the end of my first year of living on oxygen full time, 24 hours around the clock. Doctors refer to patients with lung problems as "lungers," and COPD (chronic obstructive pulmonary disease) are the initials that capture the whole disastrous Pandora's box of lung ailments. For me, the bottom line is severe emphysematous COPD and I find it simpler just to say I have emphysema.

I have been in active combat with the ailment for approximately 10 years. In fact, the beginning warnings were so long ago that I can hardly remember when I could walk up a steep hill, slide across a dance floor, or chase after small children. I do not have the horrendous cough frequently associated with the disease, but I am continuously oxygen starved and I can feel this condition from my head to my toes. I do not mind so much that my feet are numb most of the time, but every now and then it does occur to me to wonder what might be happening to my brain.

I have been hospitalized 7 times in the past 3 years with one of the visits a 3-day stay in an ICU unit. Of course, there are the continuous monthly checkups, the blood gas tests, the fine tuning, so to speak, and I am fortunate to be in the care of some of the best doctors in the country. I have a close association, and a considerable file, with my friend, the druggist. Blue-Cross-Blue Shield communicates with me almost daily and I'm grateful for their participation in my problem. The medications that help you breathe are expensive and some of them may also have some unpleasant side effects. But everything is a trade-off and when you find yourself slowly smothering day after day after day, there is a tendency to panic and an instinct to sit down quietly in some dark corner.

The condition of your lungs affects the whole person *and it's the disastrously fast disabling quality of this illness that is probably most distressing. You simply cannot believe that you can be reduced from an active independent person to a slow-moving zombie with very little chance of ever recovering your previous mobility. You have come to a lonely place in the road. But there is oxygen and what a blessing it is. It not only makes a daily routine of whatever chores you are capable of doing, but it provides some let up in the agony it is to breathe when you are having a particularly stressful day. For whatever the reasons, some days are more difficult than others. Oxygen also has a spirit-lifting quality that will allow you to get out into the world of normal people—away for awhile from your confinement and a chance to change your perspective.*

For a long time I was hesitant to appear in public with my "hose" on. Disabled people who are in wheelchairs, or who wear neck braces, or casts, or push walkers around don't even raise an eyebrow. But fit a piece of plastic into your nose and even in this sophisticated world the double takes make you feel that you have drifted in from a faraway planet. Despite my husband's encouragement, it took me quite awhile to make my first public appearance—and how vain and how foolish I was about it—and how fearful. But now the plastic hose is as much a part of my costume as my underwear and I've been thinking about designer cannulas. Surely Gucci or Pucci or Gloria Vanderbilt ought to be able to make a clever contribution, perhaps combined with an eye shade to cover puffy eyes on days when the breathing is especially tight. Of course, you cannot do anything without your doctor's permission and advice but how exciting it is to get out of your house—even if only for short periods of time.

Getting the right oxygen setup is also a matter that must fit your particular circumstances. I am most fortunate in that my husband is very handy and knowledgeable in coping with the tanks and equipment and he keeps me provided with a system that is virtually foolproof. At home I have a concentrator made in Denver, Colorado. It uses filter beds to remove nitrogen from the air and produces low-pressure oxygen which is regulated by a typical flow meter. At the rate of 4 liters per minute, it produces 96% oxygen. It weighs approximately 130 pounds and costs $2500. (Newer units weigh as little as 29 pounds.—Editor) *Medicare and hospital insurance will participate in the cost or rental. Mine has approximately 14,000 hours on it, is 2 years old, and we have it checked out once a year at the factory. It is truly a marvelous machine. I have a hose attached to it long enough to allow me to travel most everywhere around our house. Also, in the house, as an emergency source in case of a power outage, we keep two K bottles and they are also used to fill two smaller carrying bottles. A K bottle holds over 6,000 liters and my husband keeps a regulator attached for my use.* (K bottles are about the same size as H bottles.—Editor)

When I am out of the house I have a standard S bottle with a regulator on it behind the front seat of the car.

It holds approximately 4,200 liters and will last a little over 20 hours set at 3 liters. This I use for driving around. For getting out and shopping or having lunch I have a 406-liter aluminum bottle. It is about 2 feet tall, 4 inches in diameter, and weighs approximately 14 pounds when full. It comes with a carrying case and a shoulder strap and will last up to 2 hours set at 3 liters per minute. Then there's "Fatty," my favorite. Fatty is a 40-cubic foot oxygen bottle that my husband mounted on a suitcase carrier, the same as those used by airline stewardesses. It has rubber tired wheels on it and a reinforced frame. It weighs 25 to 30 pounds when full but, because of its sturdy construction, it is well balanced and easy to pull. It also makes you feel very secure, as it will last approximately twice as long as the small carrying bottle. I never go anywhere without "Fatty." (This setup was devised by her husband and worked well.—Editor)

Liquid oxygen is not yet available in our town but I have heard many good things about it. So there are all kinds of setups—roads to maintain your independence as far as your lungs will allow. Needless to say, it is most important not to take chances, to try to do things beyond your capacity on a day that is difficult and stressful.

I think it is important to realize that many people just can't be comfortable around a health problem that isn't normal. I have felt people back away from me simply because they really didn't know what to say—and their action is not meant unkindly at all. Many people are not familiar with oxygen and its uses except in emergency situations. A short time ago I made an appointment at Mr. Henri's Beauty Salon to get my hair done. I had never been there before and when I showed up with Fatty I was escorted past the hairdryer brigade to a booth. Within 2 minutes Mr. Henri himself was at my side solicitous and concerned. Would the ladies who smoked bother me? And, delicately phrased, but an obvious concern, was there any possible hazard from my tank? Mr. Henri reminded me somewhat of our airlines. After making a survey of all the major carriers, we realized that it would really be easier to board a

*plane with an atomic bomb in one hand rather than a
bottle of oxygen.*

*And then there was the lady who felt so sorry for me
that her litany of pity went on and on ending with, "You
poor dear, think of everything you can't do anymore."
"Ah ha," I said, "think of everything I don't have to do
anymore," and I thought of the heavy vacuum cleaner
or six or eight sacks of groceries to haul into the house,
even of the unwaxed kitchen floor.*

*I can think of no worse occupation than sitting around
feeling bereft of all one's best shots in life. An illness
upsets not only the patient but all those close to him—
those who care and want desperately to help. Their
days are not always so swell either and it takes lots
of love and sharing and toughing it out to come slowly
to the realization that just because the physical plant is
not functioning too well, the spirit can still soar. There
are no spare parts for the lungs but there can be pure
joy in finding you can walk a little farther than you
thought you could—that you made it through a tough
day—that, maybe, you weren't as disagreeable as you
were yesterday. (See Lung Transplantation, Chapter 8.)
You need time alone—time to get gathered together, to
renew the patience that sometimes seems to slip away
and leaves you feeling defeated and frustrated. It's okay
to be slow—there's no important race to run. There are
many new activities you can be part of, and always
there are people worse off than yourself, where you
could try to be helpful. Last year I got involved in
reading to some older residents of our nursing home, an
activity I really enjoyed, particularly Millie's reaction
to my appearance. The first week when I showed up
with Fatty she said nothing but she had a piercing look
in her eye and the next week she was waiting for me.
"Say, Lady," she chirped, "when are you going to shave
off that mustache?"*

*The young and the old, the sick and the well, we all
have something to contribute to each other. We get better
at it as time goes on and we learn to cope with our
particular situation. This miraculous flesh and blood
body we live in needs help from the best that medical
science can give us. But it also takes a guiding faith*

beyond medicine that many of us have never called upon before. This is our chance, our growth, our grace. Fatty and I plan to make the most of it. (She did indeed. This adventurous and courageous woman lived and enjoyed life for six full years after starting oxygen. Her death was from lung cancer, also related to smoking.— Editor)

New Developments in Home Oxygen Therapy

Some patients are concerned about the cosmetics of oxygen therapy. Even the double nasal cannulae illustrated in Figures 29–34 and the liquid portable system or tank create, in the mind of the patient, such an unusual appearance that he/she begins to abandon social activities outside the home. How sad, when it is well known that oxygen can extend both the length and quality of life.

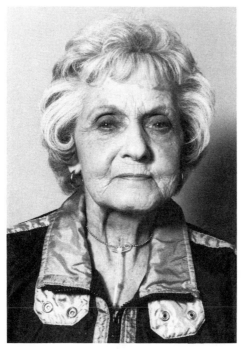

Figure 35. Use of transtracheal oxygen delivery: The oxygen flows directly into the trachea (windpipe).

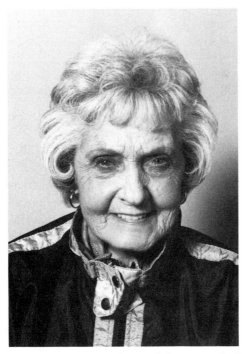

Figure 36. **Near concealment** of the transtracheal catheter is achieved by buttoning the patient's collar.

The cost of oxygen therapy is another concern, as is convenience. Thus, research has focused on cosmetics, conservation, and convenience.

One of the most novel advances includes placing a small oxygen tube directly into the windpipe (trachea). This technique, popularized by an adventurous surgeon, Dr. Henry Heimlich of Cincinnati, allows for the complete concealment of oxygen under a scarf or buttoned shirt (Figures 35, 36, and 37). Using the oxygen this way also reduces the necessary liter flow by approximately 50%. Our studies indicate that, in certain patients requiring more than 3, 4, or 5 liters of oxygen a minute, much more efficient oxygenation can be achieved via such technology. There is little question that these patients will benefit from transtracheal oxygen therapy (see selected references). The role of transtracheal

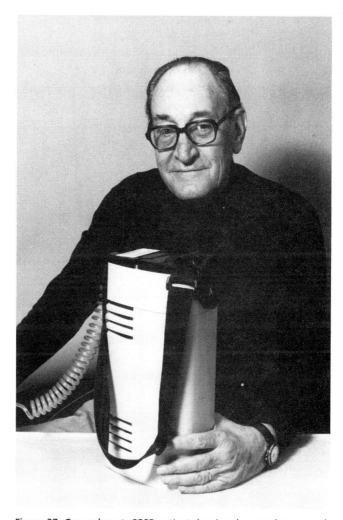

Figure 37. Concealment: COPD patient showing the complete conceal-ment of the SCOOP catheter. He is using the companion liquid portable oxygen device.

oxygen in patients requiring the more common 1 to 2 liters of oxygen per minute remains to be determined.

Demand inspiratory flow control systems are becoming in-creasingly popular. These devices allow for the flow of oxygen only during inspiration, conserving oxygen during exhalation. These devices help conserve oxygen and give the patient a greater duration of oxygen from smaller containers while away from home.

Further conservation of oxygen would allow for the manufacture of lighter and perhaps even the ultimate, a portable oxygen concentrator. It is theoretically possible to make oxygen concentrators that will weigh less than 20 pounds. Thus, it is now possible that a truly portable concentrator, powered by batteries, will be developed in the foreseeable future.

The story of long-term home oxygen therapy for COPD patients, which covers the past 30 years, is an exciting chapter in medical research. Long-term oxygen is now being given to approximately 800,000 people in North America alone, with great safety and success. When medical science can improve both the length and quality of life, research efforts are well rewarded.

As stated earlier, by no means do all patients with emphysema or COPD require oxygen, but it is useful and highly effective for selected patients with advanced COPD. It must be prescribed by your doctor. In properly selected patients, oxygen extends life and improves the quality of life. It is safe and reasonably convenient. Thus, the establishment of oxygen therapy in the care of certain patients with advanced emphysema can be considered a real advance in the story of improved health care for segments of our society.

Suggested Reading

Scientific:

1. Nocturnal Oxygen Therapy Trial Group: Continuous or nocturnal oxygen therapy in hypoxemic chronic obstructive lung disease (a clinical trial). Ann Intern Med 1980; 93:391–398.

2. Petty TL: Prescribing Home Oxygen for COPD. New York, Thieme-Stratton, 1982.

3. Petty TL: Ambulatory Oxygen. New York, Thieme-Stratton, 1983.

4. Petty TL: Pulmonary rehabilitation—Better living with new techniques. Respiratory Care, 1985;30:98–107.

5. Petty TL: Home Oxygen Therapy. Mayo Clin Proc 1987; 62:841–847.

6. Christopher KL, Spofford BT, Petrun MD, et al: A program for transtracheal oxygen delivery; assessment of safety and efficacy. Ann Intern Med 1987;107:802–808.

Report of Oxygen Consensus Conferences (which dealt with prescribing and reimbursement issues):

1. Summary of a Conference on Home Oxygen Therapy held in Denver, February 28 and March 1, 1986. Problems in prescribing and supplying oxygen for Medicare patients. Am Rev Respir Dis 1986;134:340–341.

2. Summary of the Second Conference on Long-term Oxygen Therapy held in Denver, Colorado, December 11–12, 1987. Further recommendations for prescribing and supplying longer-term oxygen therapy. Am Rev Respir Dis 1988;138:745–747.

3. Summary of the Third Consensus Conference held in Washington, DC, March 15–16, 1990. New problems in supply, reimbursement, and certification of medical necessity for long-term oxygen therapy. Am Rev Respir Dis 1990;142:721–724.

4. Further Recommendations Concerning Prescribing, Reimbursement, Technology Development, and Research in Long Term Oxygen Therapy (LTOT). Am Rev Respir and Crit Care Med, 1994;150:865–869.

CHAPTER SEVEN

PULMONARY REHABILITATION

Patients with advanced chronic pulmonary disease are primarily disabled because of shortness of breath (dyspnea). They may also be disabled by the psychological reaction to shortness of breath. These people's conditions may greatly improve with simple measures aimed at rehabilitation.

What is Rehabilitation for COPD?

The official definition of pulmonary rehabilitation is "an art of medical practice wherein an individually tailored, multidisciplinary program is formulated which, through accurate diagnosis, therapy, emotional support, and education stabilizes or reverses both the physio- and psychopathology of pulmonary diseases and attempts to return the patient to the highest possible functional capacity allowed by his pulmonary handicap and overall life situation." This statement was published in 1974 by a Committee of the American College of Chest Physicians chaired by Thomas L. Petty.

How can these goals be translated into benefits for you, the patient?

First, patients with COPD need to understand shortness of breath, a result of abnormal lung mechanics. The nonelastic lung does not empty well, and air passages, clogged with inflammation and mucus, resist airflow. These air passages also collapse, since they are not supported by the elastic tissue that helps pull them open. To compensate for this lack of elasticity, the patient's lungs expand outward to exert a little more pull on conducting air passages and increase airflow. This causes the chest to become ballooned out or to create the so-called "barrel chest."

Over-inflation puts the breathing muscles at a mechanical disadvantage. The main breathing muscle, or diaphragm, normally curved so it can descend as it contracts, is flattened from over-inflation of the lungs. Also, the muscles between the ribs are shortened, so that further contraction is difficult. Thus, the respiratory muscles are in the inflation position *before* the breathing effort begins, and cannot generate much additional force for inspiration.

The mere act of leaning forward helps to reverse this state of over-inflation. Leaning forward tends to relax the diaphragm and also reduces its troublesome reflexes. Thus, bending forward improves lung capacity. With improved lung capacity and relaxation of the breathing muscles, as well as suppression of the abnormal reflexes, shortness of breath is often reduced or eliminated.

Breathing Retraining and Exercises

The next rehabilitation procedures are breathing retraining and breathing exercises. Breathing retraining focuses on controlled diaphragmatic action; it may be taught with the patient in a seated or supine position and the therapist or nurse extending pressure on the diaphragm (Figure 38). Placing a light-weight sand bag or a heavy book on the abdomen may also help the patient concentrate on diaphragmatic breathing. This pressure on the belly muscles also tends to overcome hyperinflation and reduce abnormal reflexes in the shortened diaphragm. These techniques can relieve shortness of breath. Figure 39 (on page 98) shows a group of patients seated on pads, practicing abdominal diaphragmatic breathing with exhalation against pursed lips.

When the patient is in the upright position, the belly must bulge out during inspiration. This posture allows for the diaphragm to descend. The protuberant belly is augmented by leaning forward. Exhalation should be done through pursed lips. The technique of blowing out against slightly pursed lips, as in the act of whistling, is illustrated in Figure 40. It causes one to contract the abdominal musculature, thereby forcing the diaphragm upward to empty the lungs more

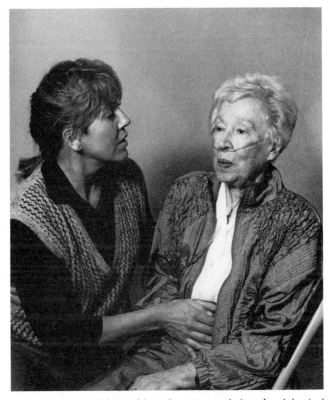

Figure 38. Abdominal Breathing: The correct technique for abdominal diaphragmatic breathing. COPD patients should relax accessory muscles and breathe with the belly, contracting abdominal muscles during expiration to help empty the lungs. The abdomen should be relaxed and become protuberant during the act of inspiration, and contract to help empty the lungs on expiration. The respiratory therapist, left, is feeling the relaxation (inspiratory) and contraction (expiratory) phases of abdominal diaphragmatic breathing.

completely. Breathing out against the resistance of pursed lips also slows respiration and thus encourages better emptying of the lungs or, in short, more efficient breathing. Thus, the combination of leaning forward, slow controlled abdominal breathing, and exhaling against pursed lips really works in reducing shortness of breath.

Patients can actually strengthen their respiratory muscles by breathing against resistance, as in pursed-lip breathing.

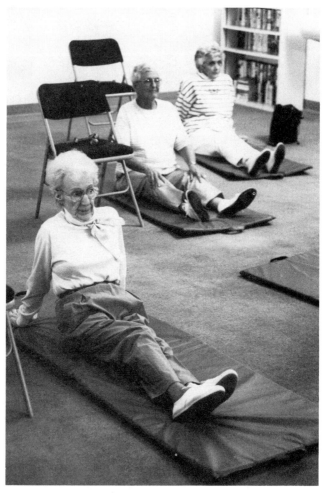

Figure 39. Practicing: COPD patients practicing controlled abdominal-diaphragmatic breathing while seated on a floor mat.

Theophylline, often used as a bronchodilator for COPD, helps strengthen the breathing muscles (see Chapter 5). Systemic exercise also strengthens the muscles and respiration. Each patient should plan to walk at least 20 minutes twice a day. Increasing each exercise period is also a good exercise strategy. Walking for 45–60 minutes once a day will help maintain good physical conditioning.

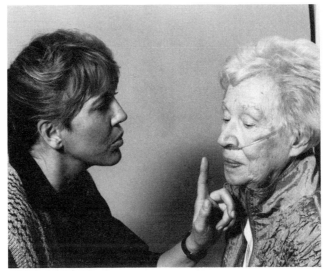

Figure 40. Pursed Lips: Patient learning proper technique of pursed lip breathing.

Although devices to promote "breathing exercises" have been presented, we continue to believe that ordinary walking and participation in regular activities of daily living are the best "breathing exercises." (See below)

Some of the exercise techniques that have been regularly employed by the pulmonary rehabilitation program at Denver's Lutheran Hospital under the direction of Judy Tietsort, RN, with the medical assistance of Dennis Clifford, MD, and with respiratory and physical therapists Brenda Crowe and Judy Tietsort, are illustrated in Figures 41–46. This program was patterned after the University of Colorado program initiated by the authors in 1966.

Another excellent program is directed by Mary Burns at Little Company of Mary Hospital in California. These facilities helped the Pulmonary Education and Research Foundation of Lomita, California, develop a tape entitled the "Essentials of Pulmonary Rehabilitation." Copies of the tape and its accompanying booklets are available through

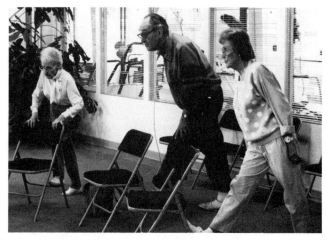

Figure 41. **Three patients** warming up with stretching exercises. One of these patients is receiving transtracheal oxygen (man in center).

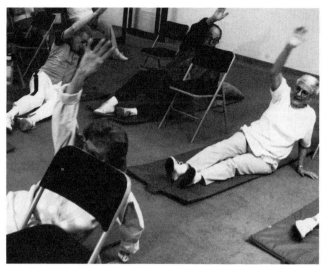

Figure 42. **Stretching:** The techniques of stretching and loosening up arm muscles while sitting on a floor mat.

most pulmonary rehabilitation programs. A limited supply is available through the authors.

Much has been written about exercise training as part of pulmonary rehabilitation. Once patients learn breathing

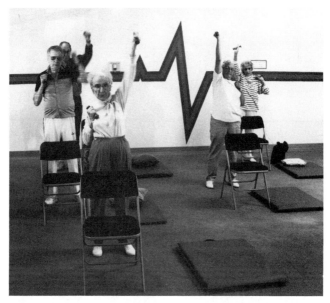

Figures 43 and 44. Exercising: Patients demonstrate attention to exercising the upper extremities. Use of the upper extremities is commonly associated with increased dyspnea, so training in this area is important.

and training exercises and strengthen their respiratory muscles through mild exercise, they usually can tolerate walks of increased distance each day. Normal walking is better than any other exercise and is far better than bicycle riding. Stationary bicycles, however, are useful during bad weather.

Doctors often use treadmills and exercise bicycles for research purposes, but they offer no particular advantage to patients. Thus, walking around the house, out of doors, or in heated malls during cold weather is desirable. Patients should walk at least 20 to 30 minutes twice daily. The training for a patient with COPD is much like that of an athlete: The more you exercise, the better you feel and the more shortness of breath subsides. Many patients can overcome shortness of breath with breathing training, breathing exercises, and daily walking according to a regular schedule.

Patients must realize that mild to moderate shortness of breath is not harmful. It doesn't strain the lungs or heart.

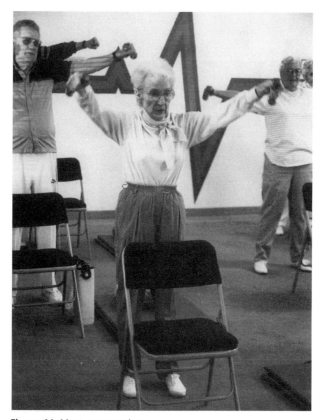

Figure 44. More arm exercises.

Many people think otherwise. They feel that if they do not overdo and take it easy, they will enjoy life more. Nothing can be further from the truth. By doing nothing, the patient with COPD eventually experiences shortness of breath during almost every activity. A vicious cycle develops. We call this the dyspnea (shortness of breath) spiral (see Figures 47 & 48). More inactivity leads to more shortness of breath, even with mild activity. This cycle can be eliminated through breathing training, breathing exercise, and muscular conditioning.

There is much more to pulmonary rehabilitation, however, than breathing training, breathing exercises, and physical conditioning. To enjoy life with emphysema and other forms

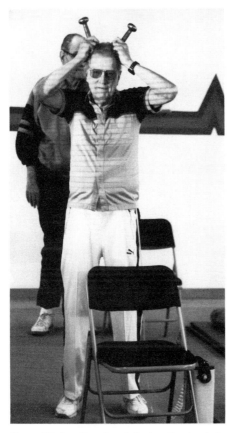

Figure 45. Arm Exercise: Patient resting bar bells on his head during exercise of arms.

of COPD, one must cope with all the problems caused by the disease. This requires the combined use of medications (see Chapter 5) and oxygen, if necessary (see Chapter 6). But even more importantly, the patient must develop methods for coping with shortness of breath and must understand how this symptom affects his or her entire being. Some of the psychological responses to shortness of breath and the fatigue that accompanies it are illustrated in Figure 47. The individual patient may or may not experience all of these responses. This illustration, while helpful, is a gross oversimplification of the interplay of physical and psychological factors operating in advanced COPD.

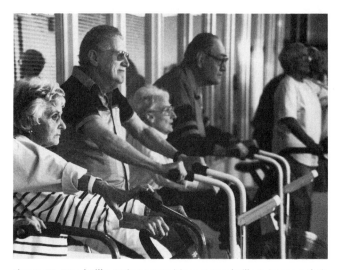

Figure 46. Treadmills: Patients exercising on treadmills to improve their exercise tolerance. (Treadmills are not seen.)

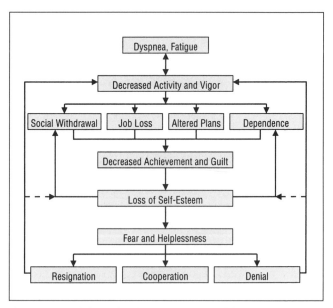

Figure 47. Psychological pathways and some of the interrelated social and symptom complexes that are consequences of severe breathing difficulties in advanced COPD.

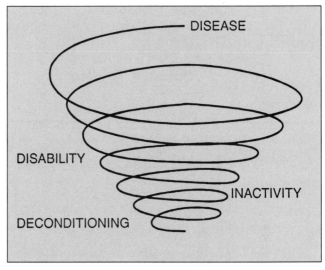

Figure 48. Downward Spiral: Symbolic representation of the downward spiral that progressively restricts the level of activity tolerated by patients with advancing COPD. Adapted from Casaburi R: Chapter XVI – Exercise Training in Chronic Obstructive Lung Disease, Casaburi R and Petty TL: *Principles and Practice of Pulmonary Rehabilitation.* WB Saunders, Philadelphia, PA 1993.

Today, more than a million patients with COPD receive Social Security benefits for disability. COPD is the most rapidly growing disability problem in the United States, ranking second behind arthritis. Many individuals with COPD would not be disabled if they had followed simple exercise training programs supplemented by breathing training, breathing exercises, and general physical conditioning.

At first, some patients can exercise only with the aid of oxygen. Those who require oxygen constantly find that they can exercise much better with oxygen than without it. The use of oxygen is covered in detail in Chapter 6.

We have rarely seen a patient who couldn't improve with instruction, training, and physical conditioning. Pulmonary rehabilitation does require determination and motivation. Becoming functional again, however, is a wonderful payoff and is the basis for really enjoying life. Being able to exercise, at least to some degree, is fundamental for work, recreation, travel, and sexuality, the subjects of later chapters in this book.

Suggested Reading

Scientific:

1. Casaburi R, Petty TL: Principles and Practice of Pulmonary Rehabilitation. W.B. Saunders, Philadelphia, PA, 1993.

Non-scientific:

1. Dewey, Jackie. Of Life and Breath. New York. Warner Books, 1986.

2. Shayevitz MB and Shayevitz BR: Living Well With Emphysema and Bronchitis. New York, Doubleday, 1985.

CHAPTER EIGHT

LUNG TRANSPLANTATION

One of the most exciting developments in the field of chronic respiratory disease states is lung transplantation. The techniques of both single and double lung transplantation have now been well established. Single lung transplantation is generally performed for patients with common forms of emphysema related to smoking and in the scarring disease known as interstitial pneumonitis with fibrosis. Single lung transplantation is a much less complex surgical procedure than double lung transplantation. Use of single lungs also serves two patients rather than one; a shortage of donor organs remains a major problem.

Problems with these procedures include infection and rejection of the transplanted lungs. Powerful drugs, critical for successful outcomes in lung transplantation, blunt the immune response and prevent rejection. These drugs also reduce the body's defenses against common infections such as viruses and bacteria, as well as fungi, which we inhale in our daily lives. Careful surveillance of infection is important in lung transplantation patients.

Double lung transplantation is reserved for patients who have serious infections of the lung at the time of transplantation. This includes all patients with cystic fibrosis, bronchiectasis, and the rare patient who can be transplanted after a period of mechanical ventilation for respiratory failure. Virtually all patients who have been on long-term mechanical ventilation have lungs that are either colonized or infected with common bacteria. The risk of infection in the transplanted lung is a real concern in these instances. A recovered transplant patient is seen in

Figure 49 with the author (TLP) and sitting at his desk at work in Figure 50.

Selecting patients for these procedures is somewhat difficult since even patients with advanced emphysema can enjoy a good quality of life for many years via home oxygen therapy and careful management. Thus, these patients may well live a decade or more without transplantation. They may be older, and transplantation is more likely to be successful in younger individuals. By contrast, patients with rapidly progressive, inflammatory, scarring lung diseases, the interstitial pneumonitis with fibrosis group, may have such a rapidly progressive disease that they lose the "window of opportunity" to receive a transplant before death ensues.

In general, patients are candidates for lung transplantation if they are under the age of 60, no longer smoke, and do not have any other major organ system disease or a recent history of any form of cancer. These patients should already have received oxygen and other potent drugs, such as bronchodilators and corticosteroids, to reverse or help stem the course of the underlying lung disease. Actually, the use of corticosteroids presents somewhat of a dilemma because corticosteroids may interfere with wound healing at the transplant site. In general, patients can receive a lung transplant if they are receiving no more than 10–15 mg daily of prednisone or its equivalent.

A regimen of pulmonary rehabilitation is required both before and after lung transplantation. At the present time, the survival rate in lung transplantation is about 80% at one year, which is an outstanding success rate compared with times past. The long-term survival effect remains to be seen, but large numbers of patients with lung transplants are now living happy and healthy lives, without serious signs of infection or rejection. Many of these patients have lived ten years or more.

While a few will be fortunate enough to be selected for this modern miracle, the treatment of advanced chronic respiratory disorders will never rest with lung transplantation because of limited organ availability, cost, and the

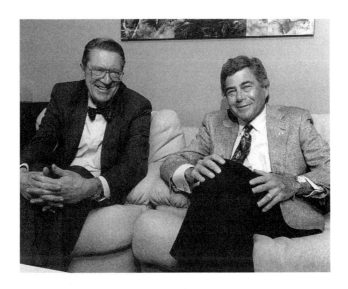

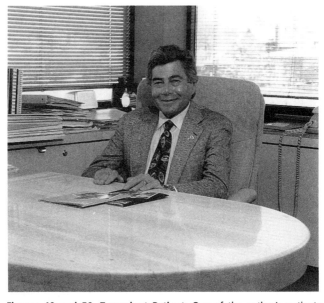

Figures 49 and 50. Transplant Patient: One of the author's patients who received a double lung transplant after a period of mechanical ventilation for acute and chronic respiratory failure. This dramatic surgery was performed by Dr. Joel Cooper and his associates at Barnes Hospital in St. Louis in March, 1993. The patient has made a complete recovery and has returned to both work and play—these pictures were taken in his office on a busy work day!

co-existent diseases that are common to many patients, including older patients. The true solution to chronic respiratory insufficiency is early identification and treatment at the first sign of cough, shortness of breath, wheeze, or any airflow abnormality.

CHAPTER NINE

WORK

The previous chapters of this book set the stage for a discussion about enjoying life with COPD. These first chapters were intended to inform the patient about COPD and how it is treated with drugs, sometimes oxygen, and pulmonary rehabilitation. Since one of the major enjoyments in life is productive work, and since coping with shortness of breath may interfere with work, a brief chapter on this topic is appropriate. (Recreation is also affected. See Chapter 10.)

Anxiety and Depression

Patients with COPD are often sad about their disease; sometimes, in fact, they are scared stiff. They may have seen other people suffer from COPD or may have heard about their problems with coping. If this is your reaction to COPD, you may prefer to close your eyes in hopes that the disease will go away. You may get depressed about your illness, since it will change your life forever. You may be irritable and angry. You turn people off. You turn yourself off. You can't sleep, you lose your appetite, you wake up in the middle of the night full of all kinds of thoughts, and you are blue. This is depression.

Our studies and those of our colleagues have indicated that high levels of depression, anxiety, and preoccupation with bodily functions occur in patients with emphysema or chronic bronchitis. We have conducted extensive psychological tests that indicate that there is not much wrong with the thinking ability of patients with COPD, but there is an identifiable pattern of psychological reactions to the disease state. The exact basis for the depression isn't exactly known, but, naturally, when people are preoccupied with breathing, they do not have enough energy for work or recreation. In addition, the exquisite complexity of the human brain is hampered by oxygen deficiency or CO_2 buildup. This problem, of course, is only present in more advanced cases and can be handled fairly well with the use of oxygen, which will correct at least part of the problem.

Our theory is that the damaged lung is failing in its role of regulating other parts of the body (Chapter 1). After all, the lung is a hormonal organ and impaired lung function can change one's mood. A change in mood, however, can result from many conditions. For example, patients who are more active are often in a better mood. Maybe this reaction is psychological, but it may also involve more than that.

We know that runners reach a "high" after heavy exertion because endorphins, natural opiates that make people feel better, are released in the brain. Recent evidence suggests that these opiates can be increased in patients with COPD through increased activities of daily living, which include exercise of both body and mind during work and recreation. Therefore, the techniques of pulmonary rehabilitation become the techniques for coping with anxiety and depression, as well as shortness of breath. Our studies have demonstrated that anxiety, depression, and preoccupation with bodily functions can be significantly improved through pulmonary rehabilitation.

Work Enjoyment

The human spirit must express its creativity through all forms of work, including manual labor, factory work, management, professional pursuits, art, music, housework—everything that is creative has value. Since work is so important to our feeling of well-being and usually is necessary to our subsistence, it is important to maintain an ability to work as long as possible. Learning to cope with shortness of breath and practicing energy-saving techniques allows people to work much longer.

We simply must expunge the idea that early retirement will somehow preserve your health and happiness. In general,

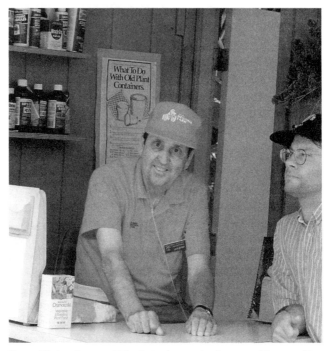

Figure 51. Landscaper: This photo shows a landscape architect working in his nursery. He is also a "plant doctor," i.e., an expert on plant diseases. Notice that he is receiving oxygen. Not shown is his portable liquid oxygen system, which contains approximately a 9-hour supply, sufficient for a full day's work. Most patients with advanced COPD who require oxygen are still able to participate in gainful employment, at least in jobs that require only sedentary activities.

the longer you work, the longer you'll be happy. We are concerned about—in fact opposed to—the growing tendency of some to advise early retirement for people with only mild to moderate impairments. In so doing, we are not only losing valuable employees, but we are also sentencing many people to years of unfulfillment and depression.

Fortunately, many employers recognize the value of keeping people in their jobs even if their productivity might plateau or even decrease. After all, it costs a lot to train new people, and replacing a valued worker costs more than just the training of a replacement. Often, the entire job environment must be adjusted when new people are hired, and new interpersonal relationships, trusts, and hopes must be established.

Oxygen therapy (see Chapter 6) should also be viewed as valuable in helping the impaired worker maintain employment. (See Figure 51.) Many of our patients have continued working for as long as a decade while using portable or stationary oxygen systems.

Some people, however, struggle at work too long and push themselves too hard. Perhaps they find work unfulfilling or frustrating. Maybe they get more satisfaction through recreational and social pursuits. They may be financially independent and want to travel or engage in hobbies. The true wishes of the patient are, at times, known only to the individual and his or her family.

In our studies, we have found that standards used to determine disability (for Social Security payments, for example) are not appropriate for many individuals. Many severely impaired candidates for retirement adapt to their jobs and do not wish to retire. Others with far less impairment simply can't continue to work, for one reason or another. The ability to maintain gainful employment does relate to the energy requirements of the job and to the individual's own physical resources. Social and psychological factors also play a role. Thus, the final decision regarding continued pursuit of one's work must be made carefully by the patient and his or her physician; hasty decisions should be avoided.

Many times, the comprehensive care and rehabilitation discussed in previous chapters of this book will help patients to work for a considerable period. Without this care, patients would be forced into early retirement.

Suggested Reading

Scientific:

1. Diener CF and Burrows B: Occupational disability patients with chronic airway obstruction. Am Rev Respir Dis 1967;96:35–42.

2. Gaensler EA and Wright GW: Evaluation of respiratory impairment. Arch Environ Health 1966;12:146–189.

3. Petty TL, MacIlroy ER, Swiger MA, and Brink GA: Chronic airway obstruction, respiratory insufficiency, and gainful employment. Arch Environ Health 1970; 21:71–78.

C H A P T E R   T E N

RECREATION

Men of age
object too much,
consult too long,
adventure too little,
and repent too soon.

FRANCIS BACON

Everyone enjoyed playing in childhood. All too often, though, opportunities for recreation during the working years are set aside because we feel a need to be productive the majority of the time. Recreation, of course, is essential in renewing one's enthusiasm for more arduous tasks, including work. In rare instances, work and recreation are synonymous. More often, we must struggle to maintain a balance between work and play.

Time for recreation is often abundant for patients with COPD. Yet recreational opportunities are not pursued by these patients, for a variety of reasons.

Major reasons include the anxiety, depression, and bodily preoccupations that permeate the minds and affect the lives and happiness of patients and their families. This triad of symptoms was discussed briefly in Chapters 2 and 9. The same problems that lead to premature abandonment of work convince patients to avoid recreation. This chapter will consider certain recreational opportunities for the patient with emphysema, but it is not an exhaustive review of every possible option. (Social interaction through COPD support groups is also described in Chapter 13.)

It is assumed that sedentary recreation will be no major problem for patients with even advanced COPD, once they can deal with their problems of mood and attitude. In fact, these problems are usually reduced after pulmonary rehabilitation begins (see Chapter 7). Reading, playing cards, watching television, and visiting with friends are recreational activities available to almost everyone.

Not so obvious are the opportunities for recreation that require increased energy expenditure through demands for increased breathing. Here too, even the patient with advanced COPD can do many things (including gardening, walking, bird watching, or people watching) by simply getting out of the house and looking past regular household activities. All too often patients fear shortness of breath, embarrassment in public, or another specific incident so much that almost all recreation is eliminated from daily life. How sad!

With improved exercise capability, discussed in Chapter 7, and improved airflow, made possible through medical measures, many patients can be much more active than they imagined possible. If these steps are not sufficient, oxygen therapy may provide just the additional boost required for happy, meaningful, and relaxing recreation. Some examples of recreational possibilities follow.

Golf

Golf does not have to be a strenuous sport. Many of our patients who were formerly competitive golfers have returned to the golf course and infused their exercise program with a little friendly competition. Even if you have no partner, you can compete against your own scores. Strolling from green to green can be paced so that almost anyone can walk through at least nine holes of play. Although golf carts are perfectly legitimate and highly useful for patients who find walking difficult (Figures 52 and 53), it is better to exercise all you can while playing golf. The breathing pattern used in exercise training is also used while walking. An inhalation of the bronchodilator just before walking up a small hill or teeing off might be enough to make the sport fun again. A

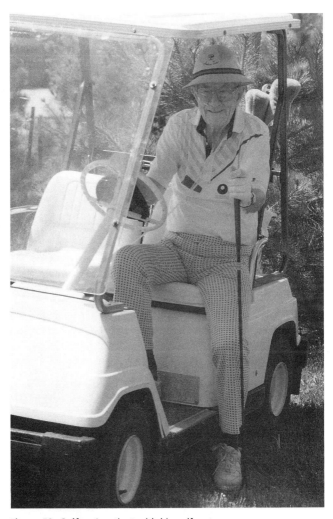

Figure 52. Golfer: A patient with his golf cart.

current patient of mine, a former "scratch golfer," still plays nine holes once a week while using oxygen.

Suppose you have never played golf. Go to a miniature golf course, practice driving, or play shortened beginners' courses. Try something new and see if you like it!

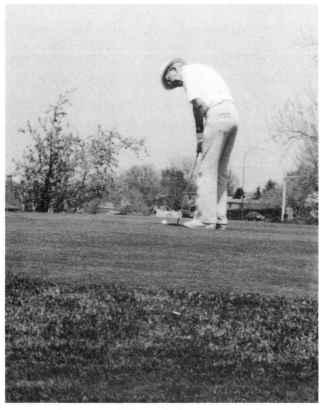

Figure 53. A patient putting on a golf green.

Bowling

Bowling does not take a lot of energy. Again, coordinate your breathing as you approach the line for a smooth swing that sends the ball on its roll down the alley. Remember, you don't need to overpower the pins. A well-placed ball is far more effective than one that swerves to the side or heads into the gutter. The weight of the ball and gravity will knock down all 10 pins if the ball is on target. Maybe you don't care to bowl at all, but you might like to go with friends while they engage in the sport. After all, somebody has to keep score!

Fishing

Fishing is easy. It's fun to fish from boats, from shore, from piers, or on ocean fishing yachts. The pleasant outdoor activity renews your energy, stimulates your appetite, and helps you sleep.

You don't have to climb up and down the banks of a Rocky Mountain stream, but even this is possible with breathing training or supplemental oxygen, when necessary. Many of our patients remain avid trout fishermen; some use small portable liquid oxygen systems.

Hunting

Many dedicated game hunters have continued to hunt on the prairie—and even travel into the mountains—with the assistance of oxygen. If hunting is impossible, spending time with a group is itself a great social outlet. You need not walk endless distances or climb high mountains in pursuit of game. Go just to smell the outdoors and the coffee!

Gardening

Gardening is a particularly fine type of recreation, available to almost everyone. Planting, watering, weeding, fertilizing, and pruning provide regular activity out of doors. Even patients with advanced COPD can partake. Figure 54 shows a patient in her favorite garden. Gardening can provide hours of recreation each day during the spring, summer, and fall.

Even if you don't have your own yard, condominiums and apartment complexes often provide areas for their residents to grow flowers or vegetables. You can also use window boxes and pots. It is particularly pleasant to watch plants grow and develop, reminding us of our own constantly changing lives.

Swimming

Many patients with COPD can engage in swimming with little shortness of breath. The buoyancy of the warm water is often quite relaxing. Even just sitting in the shallow end of the pool is fun.

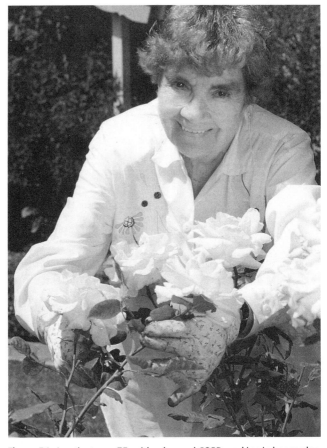

Figure 54. A patient, age 75, with advanced COPD working in her garden.

Sometimes the moist air around the pool is soothing; at other times it is not. Each individual must decide whether or not swimming is a good form of recreation. Figure 55 shows a COPD patient in a swimming pool. Notice that he is receiving oxygen via a portable liquid system placed in a flotation device.

Bicycling

Riding a bicycle is excellent exercise as well as recreation. Figure 56 illustrates how a patient with advanced COPD

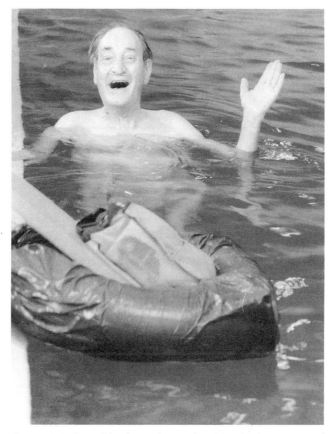

Figure 55. Patient with advanced COPD (requiring continuous oxygen) swimming in a public pool.

carries her portable liquid oxygen system in a basket attached to her bicycle.

Other Recreation Ideas

A backyard picnic, a walk through the park, or an evening of dining are simple examples of meaningful recreation. Remember that these activities require no more energy than do indoor activities at home. Unfortunately, some people avoid them for fear of shortness of breath, an attack of coughing, or just being out in crowds.

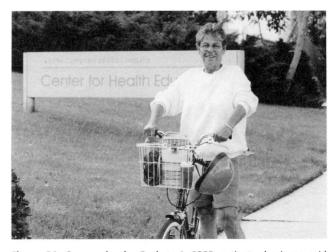

Figure 56. Oxygen in the Basket: A COPD patient who is an avid bicyclist uses oxygen carried in her bicycle basket. She rides to the hospital's pulmonary rehabilitation center to participate in activities with the patient support group. (See Chapter 13.)

It is difficult to instruct each individual reader on how to cope with their fears and anxieties. Venture forth no matter what, and do everything slowly. For some reason, patients with COPD tend to rush through all their activities, probably hoping to avoid shortness of breath if they do so. Nothing could be further from the truth. Remember the dyspnea spiral: Hurrying involves inefficient use of all muscles, including the muscles of breathing. Take your time, move slowly, do not rush, and be a bit lazy in all your activities.

This chapter ends with a plea not to abandon life and all its meaning in fear of a problem that may never come. Get up, get going, get out, and enjoy!

> *The tragedy of life is not so much what men suffer, but rather what they miss.*
>
> THOMAS CARLYLE

CHAPTER ELEVEN

TRAVEL

Travel for adventure and fun is a popular pastime in North America and other areas of the world. In fact, travel relates to other chapters of this book, including Recreation (Chapter 10), Daily Living (Chapter 14), and Remember to Live (Chapter 17). This chapter offers some specific advice about travel that may be useful to patients with serious degrees of COPD. Patients with only mild to moderate forms of disease have almost no problems with travel.

Implications of Distant Travel

When you go on a business trip or vacation, you will be separated from your medical support system, i.e., your doctor, clinic, hospital, and perhaps important medical supplies such as oxygen. In addition, the problems involved with eating in restaurants, getting in and out of hotels or motels, and changing one's daily routine are often sufficient to make traveling a low priority for many patients. This attitude is sad because travel might provide adventure, exercise that otherwise would not be pursued, and expanded horizons in life, an important principle. We feel that a realistic amount of travel is not only valuable for patients, but is almost mandatory if travel was previously part of your lifestyle.

When embarking upon a trip, of course, a supply of the usual medications required for managing your COPD is necessary. Ample supplies of inhaled and oral bronchodilators, an extra supply of corticosteroid drugs (prednisone) in case of flare-ups (see Chapter 5), and a supply of antibiotics would be appropriate. A summary of your medical history is also very useful.

If the patient with COPD really understands the disease process and knows the objectives of therapy, he or she can easily decide when a course of antibiotics should be taken (i.e., if sputum increases and is colored yellow or green, or if there is an episode of chest tightness and increased breathing difficulty that requires the additional assistance of corticosteroids) as discussed in Chapter 5. In fact, it is appropriate for the traveler to ask his or her personal physician about the most convenient time to call and discuss symptoms that may develop, any need to alter a prescribed drug regimen, or for any other advice. The physician could also give the patient the name of a contact person in a distant city from directories of qualified chest physicians, allergists, and internists.

Oxygen and Travel

Patients requiring oxygen need to make plans well in advance of their trip to ensure a continued supply. The durable medical equipment (DME) company that supplies your oxygen for home use can also assist with travel needs. It is much easier to use a company that has national offices. If you use a company other than your local supplier, you must be prepared to pay at the time of service. Be sure to keep all your paperwork for possible insurance reimbursement when you get back home. Also, bring several copies of your oxygen prescription, which you can get from your doctor or your oxygen supplier.

If you do not ordinarily use an oxygen conserving device, which can extend your time between refills by 50% to 300%, this may be the time to consider doing so. Ask your oxygen supplier about the various cannulas and oxygen-conserving containers on the market today. Some of them may change your oxygen flow and will require a specific prescription from your physician.

Travel by Car

Travel by car or van offers the most independence and mobility. The patient who needs oxygen only at night can bring along an oxygen concentrator. Request a smaller one that can be rolled on wheels like luggage. Some of these weigh about 30 pounds and can easily be stored in the trunk of the car. A porter or motel assistant can easily carry or roll the concentrator into your room just like a large suitcase.

When using liquid oxygen in the car, be sure to keep the windows cracked and the container upright. When traveling more than a day, the filling reservoir must also be taken along. Reservoirs can fit into vans, station wagons, and some larger cars. Often, your oxygen supplier can help you make adjustments in your equipment and enable you to take that special trip.

While your DME dealer may have scheduled refill stops with a 25% margin of safety, be sure to take detours, bumpy roads, and heavy traffic into consideration. Also, make sure that your refill stops use an oxygen system compatible with yours! This *should* be checked by the company planning your refills, but it is a good idea to recheck this information. If you are traveling to an area where your type of oxygen is unavailable, your company may be able to lend or rent you an adapter.

Small gas cylinders can be carried for emergency use or when driving at high altitudes. Be sure, however, that you receive written authorization from your current DME dealer for these cylinders to be refilled by another company.

Motel or hotel owners almost never refuse patients with oxygen. The public today recognizes that oxygen is not dangerous. It does not explode. It will not cause fires unless tubing is directly ignited. Reasonable precautions are all that are required before traveling with oxygen.

Pace yourself, plan stops every two hours to get out and walk, enjoy the view, and smell the flowers!

Travel By Train or Bus

Amtrak allows portable oxygen systems, including equipment weighing up to 75 pounds, on board. Advance notice of 12 hours is required. You *must* carry enough oxygen to last the entire trip, plus a safety margin of at least 20%. The wheels must be removed from wheeled containers after you are on board. Call Amtrak at 1–800–872–7245 for further information.

Greyhound Bus Lines, the only bus company serving most of the U.S., can be called at 1–800–231–2222 for information about their policies. While Greyhound allows passengers with portable oxygen on board, you may not check oxygen containers as baggage.

While many other bus lines also take passengers with oxygen and enforce no-smoking policies, it is wise to check with the individual bus company as well as the local health department or City Hall at your destination for specific information well in advance of your trip.

Travel by Sea

Ocean cruises, with their fresh sea air free from pollens and pollution, low altitude, and varied activities, can provide the ideal vacation for the person with respiratory difficulties.

Since the first cruise sponsored in 1985 by the pulmonary rehabilitation program at Little Company of Mary Hospital in Torrance, California, the number of cruise lines allowing passengers with oxygen has increased and there are few areas to which you cannot sail. However, you *must* make plans well in advance and follow the specific requirements of the line on which you wish to cruise.

If your local DME dealer does not have an office in your port of departure, they can contact another company in that area to supply your oxygen. That company will deliver your oxygen before you board and pick up the containers after you return. Bon voyage!

Travel By Plane

The pressurized cabins of modern jet aircraft maintain altitudes of 5,000 to 8,000 feet. Rarely is this range exceeded unless the airplane must fly higher to avoid weather; on these occasions, the "altitude" in the cabin can reach the equivalent of 10,000 feet.

Present regulations prohibit individuals from carrying their own oxygen systems on board, though some airlines allow *empty* oxygen systems to be checked with ordinary baggage. If you require oxygen while flying, make arrangements as far in advance as possible, though the minimum time required by most airlines is three days. Each airline requires different information that your physician will have to provide. Oxygen charges vary, but are usually a minimum of $50 for each leg of the journey. Thus, it is less costly to avoid changing planes. Also, this cost is *not* reimbursed by Medicare or any insurance policies. Oxygen provided by the airline can by used *only* on the plane. You must make additional arrangements through your oxygen supplier if you require oxygen at the airport or in transit. You should also request a wheelchair to get you to and from the plane, even if you can usually walk some distance without difficulty. Travel is stressful, so save your energy for the fun parts of it!

Thus, it is possible to travel essentially anywhere in the United States while receiving oxygen. Many of our patients have traveled from coast to coast and to Hawaii or Europe, all the while using continuous oxygen as part of their comprehensive care plan.

Let's go back to the important subject of expanding one's horizons in daily life. Visiting new areas of the country or world and reviewing the history and notable achievements of the area are interesting opportunities to most persons. Visiting parks and museums, attending theaters, or participating in ceremonial events are often meaningful experiences. It is wise to pick up reading material about the areas you visit along the way so you can renew the experience when you get back home. Reflecting over a pleasant, adventurous travel experience is a gratifying respite for many people.

TRAVEL HINTS FOR THE PERSON WITH COPD
Prepared by Mary R. Burns, RN, BS
Little Company of Mary Hospital
Torrance, California 90503

Travel upsets our usual pattern of breathing and oxygenation because it requires more exertion than we normally use. Also, we might be traveling into an area where there is less oxygen per square foot or more air pollution than we are accustomed to.

To minimize problems caused by air pollution:

• Travel before morning rush hours and after sunset.

• Avoid heavily traveled roads.

• Call ahead and get air quality information in the cities you plan to visit.

Altitudes Beware of altitudes higher than you can tolerate either at your destination or while traveling. Remember when flying that if necessary, a wheelchair can be brought to and from the plane and you can arrange in advance for special boarding and seating.

Temperatures Cold air can cause bronchospasm and associated shortness of breath. Avoid really frigid temperatures. Wear light but warm clothing.

Warm climates are generally preferable to cold, except when temperatures go over 90 degrees. In this case, stay inside where it is air conditioned!

Allergies First, know what you are allergic to.

• Ragweed—avoid central and eastern states in the flowering season. Go to the far west or north.

• Dust and mold—may be encountered in hotel rooms. If necessary request a room change or bring your own portable electronic air filter.

• Beware of feather pillows and comforters, especially in Europe.

Medications

- Carry duplicates in your handbag, separate from your luggage.

- Each container should be labeled with your name, the name of the medication, and the drug's strength.

- Carry a physician's summary of your current medications. This will help you through customs and also if you have to see another physician in an emergency. A physician's recent summary of your medical history and pertinent findings from his latest examination of you: Blood pressure, recent arterial blood gases if available, pulmonary function tests (FVC and FEV_1), pulse, respiratory rate, and status of your lungs and heart.

- Make friends with your pharmacist. Arrange to have him airmail you your prescription refills, rather than trying to replace them while you're out of town.

Medical Assistance Before leaving home, obtain the name of a physician at your destination. If you are going abroad, you can contact IAMAT— International Association of Medical Assistance to Travelers at 350 Fifth Avenue, Suite 5620, New York, New York 10001. This organization is familiar with North American and British medical techniques. Take along your doctor's telephone number, but remember the time changes if you call!

Oxygen

- If you are going to be traveling in an automobile, you can carry a storage unit (known as the reservoir) for your portable liquid oxygen system. It will hold a 3- to 4-day supply or more. Beware; you may travel through some areas of high altitude.

- If you will need oxygen on an airplane, you should notify the airline at least 72 hours in advance (1 week is better). You will need a written prescription from your physician certifying your need and maximum flow rate.

- There are no regulations restricting the use of your oxygen during rail travel. They do request that you notify them when you make your reservations. Again, watch your altitude.

- If you are going to be traveling on a Greyhound bus, you must sit in the No Smoking section and be self-sufficient. If you need a helper, two can ride for the price of one, but you must provide a doctor's letter stating your need.

In general, plan ahead. Carry your oxygen prescription with you and, before you leave home, obtain the name of a dealer at your destination so you can get a refill when needed.

Nebulizers

- Carry IPPBs or pump nebulizers, if you use them, with your carry-on luggage to avoid breakage.

- Bring a note from your physician explaining your respiratory equipment. This may minimize delay at security checkpoints.

- Allow enough time for your treatments.

General Problems of Travel

- *Motion Sickness*—If this is a problem, ask for Dramamine® or Marezine® before you begin your trip. Also, you should travel in the least bumpy part of the vehicle (the center of an airplane). Transderm II applied to the skin also is useful for some people with motion sickness. The active ingredient is scopolamine, related to atropine, which makes some people feel "spacey."

- *Fatigue*—Don't overexert and do get enough sleep. Plan ahead and pace yourself.

- *Jet Lag*—Your body rhythms get confused when you travel across several time zones. For COPD patients, morning is the worst time, so leave plenty of time for inhalation therapy, breathing exercises, coughing, etc. You must reestablish your daily routines.

- *Constipation*—The differences in time, diet, accommodations and relaxation patterns all take their toll and may cause irregularity. Also, gas expands in the intestines during travel; this may cause bloating and make breathing difficult. It is recommended that you take a mild roughage stimulant each morning and, if necessary, a mild bulk laxative, e.g., Metamucil®.

- *Diarrhea*—Remember that the more profuse the diarrhea, the more likely the dehydration and loss of essential minerals. Drinking bouillon, apple juice or Gatorade® is recommended. Diarrhea might be avoided by taking tablets to disinfect water and using Lomotil®, if your doctor suggests it. Pepto-Bismol® is also effective and safer than Lomotil.

- *Vomiting*—This can cause bronchospasm and prevent oral medications from being absorbed.

- *Overeating*—Avoid excessive alcohol or food intake. This can cause bloating, which uses up much-needed air space.

Before you leave home, familiarize yourself with your destination, plan the easiest way to go, and pace yourself.

Insurance Check your health insurance before you leave and carry blank forms. Blue Cross and some others will mail you a travel kit. Medicare will not cover you outside the United States, but some insurance policies do. You can also check with your travel agent about medical coverage. Trip interruption insurance might be worth considering, but it does not cover pre-existing conditions! There are many organizations you can consult for help if you are traveling overseas.

CHAPTER   TWELVE

SEXUALITY

Many people will read this chapter first. Frankly, we don't blame them, since concerns about sexuality are exceedingly common and perplexing for patients with COPD. Fortunately, many in our profession are taking a greater interest in this subject, as we have for years. Scientific programs, public forums, articles, and books about sexuality are becoming increasingly common. The suggested reading list at the end of this chapter offers further opportunity for study about the numerous and frustrating problems of sexual non-interest or sexual dysfunction in patients with all degrees of COPD. The three articles *written for everyone* are particularly recommended.

The vast majority of older people maintain some sexual interest and, at times, intense sexual desire, but some reduction in sexual interest and activity is natural as people age. This normal state can be complicated by real or perceived sexual limitations for both men and women in various stages of COPD. Many men have difficulty achieving or maintaining an erection; they may simply give up before or during sexual activity because of shortness of breath or its associated frustration. A woman may fail to "turn on" to the notion of sex or to appropriate suggestions and gestures by her partner, or may simply have little interest in sexual activity.

The solution to these problems begins with openness and understanding. The first step is often simply an acknowledgment of the problems and frustrations experienced by either partner. We always talk to our patients about this topic and patients are almost always grateful that we do.

Most patients would simply like to get their thoughts and concerns "out in the open." Perhaps just reading this portion of the book will help.

Most sexual dysfunction can be handled by a simple informative approach. Attempts at lovemaking while fatigued, during a chest infection, following a large meal, or after indulging in large amounts of alcohol are destined to fail. After all, we should be ready for something as important as sex. Being mentally out of phase with your partner's developing arousal is also a mistake. Both partners must get interested in the same thing at the same time. Most important is the principle of approaching lovemaking in a slow and deliberate manner. In fact, patients with COPD tend to do all things too quickly, probably in the mistaken belief that if they rush an activity, it will be accomplished without shortness of breath. Nothing could be farther from the truth.

Taking an inhaled bronchodilator before sexual activity is a good practice. The bronchodilator relaxes the air passages and provides improved breathing capacity. Taking oxygen before or during lovemaking may also be helpful.

Beyond these simple suggestions, sexual techniques must be discussed. Changing from the traditional position to side-by-side, woman on top, seated in a chair, and other positions to increase comfort is helpful to certain couples. Long periods of caressing and engaging in gentle mutual stimulation, self-pleasuring, and oral sex are not only quite acceptable, but can be pleasant and satisfying for many couples (though not all). We do not intend to change any patient's sexual practices, and certainly we do not try to make major changes in sexual attitudes. Rather, we aim to encourage all of our patients and their mates to investigate and adventure on behalf of their mutual happiness. More frequently than not, couples are delighted at the "permission" to explore. Many times they have been bound by inhibitions rooted in the past. Understanding the broad range of "normalcy" is reassuring. Any sexual activity that is naturally pleasing and satisfying is, of course, "normal" activity. "If it feels right, do it," we advise.

Most of all, we encourage tenderness in all aspects of life. After all, sexual activity isn't just the "main event." Kind words, hand holding, touching, and hugging are fulfilling experiences for all of us.

Sex and the Lungs

Probably the most damaging factors in the avoidance or failure of sexual expression by patients with COPD (no matter what their marital situation has been in the past) are poor self-image, fear of rejection, and fear of failure to perform and satisfy. Actually, poor self-image results from the struggle to cope with an illness that attacks the body's most fundamental organs—the lungs. This poor self-image may, however, be more than just a psychological reaction to a serious chronic illness. The lungs and their functions have an important impact on every other organ of the body, including the sex organs. Not much is known about the function of the testes, ovaries, or the ancillary reproductive organs in the presence of oxygen shortage or carbon dioxide build-up. However, since every cell of the body, including the organs that produce sex hormones, requires oxygen for energy production, it is highly likely that lung dysfunction may directly interfere with basic sexual drives and performance. We do know that there is a reduction in male sex hormone (testosterone) in some men with COPD.

In addition, the lungs play a fundamental role in the metabolic function of other organs. The lungs process many materials that are brought to them via the venous blood and they can modify hormonal chemicals within the body, which certainly could effect sexual functioning. Furthermore, altered lung function—with or without abnormal levels of oxygen and carbon dioxide—has a great impact on brain function. Complex and integrated brain function is largely mediated by internal brain chemicals called neurotransmitters. Neurotransmitters are dependent on an adequate supply of oxygen. Thus, it can be easily understood how, with severe lung disease, sexual tranquility can be badly damaged or completely wrecked.

As sexual beings, we certainly are not just testes, ovaries, penis, and vagina, but rather an integrated system with a brain and higher centers of thinking and feeling. In fact, these are probably the most important parts of the sexual experience, apart from the necessity of reproduction to sustain the human species. The importance of sexual activity lies in our ability to express love, hope, human caring, self-worth, and sharing. These feelings certainly involve finely tuned and integrated brain function, efficient lung function, and, indeed, all the functions of the body.

Overcoming Fears and Taboos

There are simple explanations for sexual fears or taboos. Many times patients fear that any form of sexual activity will be too exhausting, too stressful to the heart, or somehow damaging to the lungs or other organ systems. Sexual activity, well performed, is almost never exhausting and is not too stressful for people with even severe impairments of lungs and heart. You will suffer no harm and will not harm your lover through any form of sexuality. It is not dangerous to love and adventure.

We believe that individuals place too many restrictions on themselves and their attractiveness to others. Thus, the concept of one's self as a sexual being who is attractive to another person is distorted, damaged, or destroyed. Barriers become established after years of frustration and self-doubt. These attitudes must be replaced through counseling.

Howard Kravetz[1] of Prescott, Arizona has been one of the pioneers in explaining the sexual problems of men and women who suffer from COPD. Kravetz and his associates have produced a slide-tape presentation that has been widely hailed by members of the American College of Chest Physicians and the American Thoracic Society as something valuable for those who suffer from emphysema and other forms of COPD.

Also, Dr. Paul Selecky of Newport Beach, California, is an expert in human sexuality and the COPD patient. We

---

[1]Present address: 1011 Ruth Street, Prescott, AZ 86301

recommend his chapter in a recently released textbook on pulmonary rehabilitation. (See Suggested Reading list at the end of this chapter.)

In brief, the experts' message is simple. It is based on an understanding of the reasons for lack of sexual interest or functioning. Both Kravetz and Selecky recommend, as we do, a simple straightforward solution to the problem based on the willingness of both partners to experiment in some form of loving sexual activity. This need not be full expression of the sexual act. Hand holding, then hugging, caressing, fondling, stroking, and, finally, more intimate forms of sexual interaction are advised. It takes initiative, a bit of an adventurous spirit, and certainly a great deal of patience to progress through the various degrees of sexual functioning once again. The drives, urges, reflexes, abilities, and interests remain if one patiently tries to reawaken lost feelings and abilities instead of postponing hopes and desires.

We must end this chapter with another quote from the late Dr. Alvan Barach. The following poem was published in the *Columbia University Physicians and Surgeons Quarterly*:

ADVICE TO THE LOVELORN

Better live in Iwo-Jima
Than have pulmonary emphysema.
Better love fair ladies
Before you're in the eighties
(Mons veneris is a crest
But it's not Mount Everest.)
Live wild enough to keep sane
And not get old in vain.

ALVAN L. BARACH '19

We recognize that this chapter has not dealt with every aspect of the enjoyment of sexuality. It is intended to present an approach to coping with the problems of frustration and failure, and to give the reader some new ideas about how to enjoy life, including a satisfying sex life, with COPD.

Suggested Reading

Scientific:

1. Angle DP and Baum GL: Psychological aspects of chronic obstructive pulmonary disease. Med Clin North Am 1977; 61:749–758.

2. Fletcher E and Martin RJ: Sexual dysfunction and erectile impotence in chronic obstructive pulmonary disease. Chest, 1982;81:413–421.

3. Frank E, Anderson C and Rubenstein D: Frequency of sexual dysfunction in "normal" couples. N Engl J Med 1978;299:111–115.

4. Kass I, Updegraff K and Muffly RB: Sex in chronic obstructive pulmonary disease. Med Aspects of Human Sexuality 1972;6:33–42.

5. Kolodny RC, Masters H and Johnson VE: Textbook of Sexual Medicine, Boston, Little, Brown & Co., 1979.

6. Kravetz HM: Sexual counseling for the COPD patient. Clinical Challenge in Cardiopulmonary Med 1982;4:1–5.

7. Sample PD, Beastall GH and Hume R: Male sexual dysfunction, low serum testosterone and respiratory hypoxia. Br J Sexual Med 1980;13:48–53.

8. Sample PD, Beastall GH, Watson WS, and Hume R: Hypothalamic-pituitary dysfunction in respiratory hypoxia. Thorax 1981;36:605–609.

9. Zilbergeld B: Male Sexuality. Boston, Little, Brown & Co., 1978.

10. Madorsky JG, Dixon TP: Rehabilitation aspects of human sexuality. West J Med 1983;139:174–176.

11. Selecky P: Sexuality and the patient with lung disease. (In) Casaburi R, Petty TL (eds): Principles and Practice of Pulmonary Rehabilitation, Saunders, Philadelphia, 1993.

Written For Everyone (both Scientific and Non-scientific):

1. Comfort A: The Joy of Sex. New York, Crown, 1972.

2. Masters WH: Sex and Aging—Expectation and Reality. Hospital Practice, 1986;21:175–198.

3. Petty TL: Health, Sex and Better Quality of Life for Your COPD Patient. Medical Aspects of Human Sexuality. August 1986:70–85.

CHAPTER THIRTEEN

PATIENT AND FAMILY SUPPORT GROUPS

Patients with various degrees of COPD have found that the organization of support groups can be extremely helpful from many points of view. The opportunity to share experiences about coping with shortness of breath and to learn about new therapeutic advances, including drugs and devices, are obvious benefits of patient support groups. Of greater importance, however, is the opportunity to socialize in a healthy environment as one learns to live with chronic lung problems.

One of the most exciting patient support groups is the PEP Pioneers at Little Company of Mary Hospital in Torrance, California. Another is Project MOVE at Lutheran Hospital in Wheatridge, a suburb of Denver, Colorado. The PEP Pioneers consist of graduates from the pulmonary rehabilitation program at that hospital. The group's organizer, Mary Burns, RN, BS, has been the spiritual leader of the Pioneers since its inception. Their newsletter, distributed nationally, is called "PEP Pioneers—Second Wind."[1] It offers news about the PEP Pioneers themselves as well as contributions from doctors, nurses, and therapists who are on the forefront of research and care for patients with COPD.

The group's annual respiratory rally, held in the spring of each year, has become a national event. One of us (TLP) had

---

[1]Available on request—PEP Pioneers, Little Company of Mary Hospital, 4101 Torrance Blvd., Torrance, Ca 90503.

the opportunity to compete in this rally. The contest itself is a "paced race;" each individual estimates the time it will take him or her to walk the length of a marked course. The point is not speed but rather accuracy in estimating the time needed to complete the course without undue respiratory distress. Thus, if you predict that your time will be 2 minutes and you finish the course in 1 minute, obviously you fail. If, on the other hand, you predict that your walk will take 8 minutes and it takes 8 minutes and 5 seconds, you will likely be the first place winner.

This "paced race" symbolizes the necessity of controlling one's energy expenditure to complete the task required in a systematic fashion. The objective of pacing one's self throughout the activities of daily living is epitomized in this annual event. (I have to confess that I didn't do well in my first paced race. I underestimated my time and completely overestimated the necessary time for others to complete the course. On the next occasion, I will be better advised—TLP.)

Perhaps the most remarkable activity of the PEP Pioneers has been their series of pioneering ocean voyages. Through immense effort and careful planning, Mary Burns and her associates hurdled bureaucratic roadblocks and obtained clearance for a sea cruise for patients, including those requiring ambulatory oxygen, who had prematurely restricted their own horizons. These outings have become a regular activity for many support groups here and in Europe.

Several Colorado groups meet on a regular monthly basis. The format of each meeting varies, but usually includes a speaker who brings some new item of interest to the group. Most topics are medically oriented and focus on COPD. Announcements and refreshments follow the presentation and open-ended socializing completes each regular meeting. Special events such as picnics and "pot luck" dinners are also scheduled at various times throughout the year.

The excellent program at Lutheran Medical Center, under the direction of nurse-therapist Judy Tietsort, has been an inspiration to both of us. Figures 57, 58, and 59 show a few activities of the group and tell a story more eloquently than our words can.

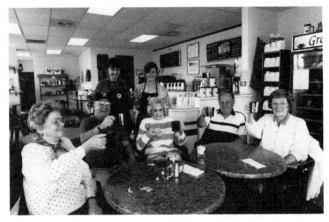

Figure 57. Patient support group at Lutheran Medical Center enjoying coffee at the pulmonary rehabilitation unit.

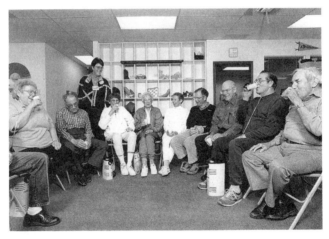

Figure 58. Respiratory therapist Brenda Crowe (standing) with patients at a "tune up" session enjoying refreshments in the pulmonary rehabilitation unit.

We always encourage our patients to join a patient support group. Such activity is rewarding for patients with even mild to moderate stages of disease. Occasionally, we detect some reluctance on the part of the patient or family when we suggest enrolling in one of these groups. Patients may initially feel some reticence to associate with "so many sick

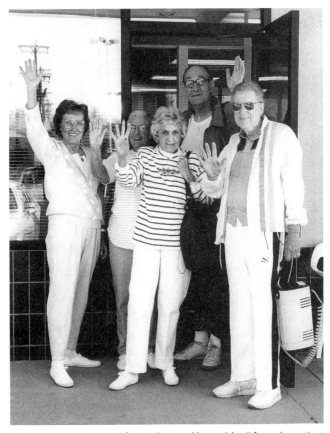

Figure 59. An expression of "greetings and best wishes" from the patient support group at Lutheran Medical Center in Wheatridge, Colorado.

people." In truth, these groups maintain a positive attitude toward enjoyment of life that helps patients realize that their fears of being consumed by progressive illness are unfounded. Also, many patients with only moderate disease recognize their own relatively good health compared to the plight of others. Even more important is seeing how well those with advanced disease can deal with the problem. This powerful testimony can later be used to cope with advanced disease if it should develop.

We recognize COPD as a progressive process, but we try to maintain stability by forestalling or reversing the course of disease. Enjoying life, having pleasant social interactions, and constantly learning through the exchange of ideas with others make the support group experience thoroughly rewarding. Participation in such groups also offers the individual the opportunity to contribute his or her own energies, experiences, and abilities to the group as a whole. Thus, the feedback, feeling of accomplishment, and constant gaining of knowledge are payoffs for those who make the necessary effort and commitment. The philosophy of the PEP Pioneers, as expressed by their leadership, is as follows: "It is a group of patients . . . whose purpose is to keep in touch, to express concern for one another's health and progress, and to continue education about their pulmonary dysfunction."

We are all "social beings." Few people can live happily and comfortably as "an island," isolated from outside social contact. Human interaction helps to release our anxieties, fears, and concerns about life and the future. It helps to keep us going—living and enjoying.

Suggested Reading

Two *Musts* for COPD Patients and Their Families:

1. PEP Pioneers Second Wind
   Little Company of Mary Hospital
   4101 Torrance Boulevard
   Torrance, California 90503
   Published Monthly

2. Essentials of Pulmonary Rehabilitation: A "Do-It-Yourself" Program.
   Part I, 1991
   Part II, 1992
   Part III, 1993
   Available free from:
   Pulmonary Research & Education Foundation (PREF)
   P.O. Box 1133
   Lomita, California 90717-5133

CHAPTER FOURTEEN

DAILY LIVING

This chapter aims to provide some general information on the details of daily living that will be of interest to many patients. Section headings identify specific topics.

Place of Residence

Many people ask us about the best climate or location for patients with COPD. It is difficult to give specific advice for each individual, because lifelong experience, the location of family and friends, church affiliations, and personal preferences are very important. In general, a location with a low altitude and mild climate would be preferable. Many people, therefore, have moved to the west coast of Florida, the gulf area, and along the gulf coast from Florida to Texas. The Southwest is also popular, primarily the greater Phoenix area. San Diego and Palm Springs, California, are other popular locations. Each of these places offers the advantage of low altitude where, of course, the most oxygen is present. These regions generally have a temperate climate and little air pollution. Inversions, which trap polluted air near the ground, are rare in the southeast because of the prevailing winds. The economics of living in these popular areas must always be considered.

The west coast of Florida and the Gulf of Mexico have essentially no air pollution. On the other hand, high humidity in these areas may be a problem for those patients who feel more shortness of breath on high-humidity days. Excessive heat can also be a problem. The heat, of course, can be overcome with air-conditioning, even in cars, but it is hardly desirable to be confined to an air-conditioned environment most of the time.

The early morning and evening hours in the desert are generally cool and quite pleasant for almost everyone. Some patients have difficulty with the pollens from desert flowers and weeds, but this problem is not usually serious. Desert dust, on the other hand, can be a more serious problem and needs to be considered if one is thinking about living in the Southwest.

The southern California coast is also quite pleasant, with very moderate temperatures. Again, humidity may be a problem. Pollution around such major cities as San Diego and Los Angeles is also troublesome to the patient with COPD. There are many pleasant areas to live north of Los Angeles, where mild climate and freedom from air pollution can be enjoyed, but the cost of living in these areas is prohibitive to many. Other places throughout the world may also offer a splendid climate and living surroundings, but problems with access to modern medical care, oxygen supplies, and other necessities of the COPD patient may exist.

Another way to learn about the "ideal" place of residence and the best weather is to be a bit peripatetic and move back and forth following the good seasons. Many of our patients in Colorado, Wyoming, and Montana enjoy the spring, summer, and fall in these regions and then travel to a warmer, more sunny climate during three or four winter months. Avoiding extreme cold is generally useful, since exposure to cold often causes some degree of bronchospasm, thereby making exercise more difficult than usual. In addition, over-chilling can reduce the body's natural defenses against viral infections, which often are the prelude to more serious bacterial infections like bacterial bronchitis or overt pneumonia.

Diet

A good diet provides both pleasure and important energy for the patient with COPD. Almost any type of food can be enjoyed by these patients, with certain limitations. Such limitations are so dependent on an individual's tolerance for food, however, that it is almost impossible to give specific advice. In general, a balanced diet that includes protein, carbohydrates, and fat, with an appropriate amount of calories to maintain an "ideal weight" is the wise rule to follow.

No particular food must be avoided unless there are specific upsets from it. Some people feel that milk products form excessive mucus, but there has never been any proof of this notion. Personally, we doubt this idea. Any food leading to allergic reactions such as rashes or other eruptions should not be eaten. Foods that create excessive gas, such as some bulky vegetables and cooked beans, are probably best avoided. Any distention of the abdomen from gastrointestinal gas can increase respiratory distress because the abdominal muscles cannot relax properly and abdominal diaphragmatic breathing is hindered (see Chapter 7). In addition, any patient who has suffered a swelling of the ankles due to edema (salt and water) formation, either with or without associated failure of the heart, should avoid excessively salty food and should refrain from using table salt. If the physician feels a patient needs a low-salt or "salt-free" diet, specific prescriptions should be offered.

Individuals need to maintain an appropriate weight. Any weight loss, unless necessary because of obesity, is a cause for concern. For some reason, patients with COPD tend to lose body weight and, finally, muscle mass in the advanced stages of their illness. The exact cause of this phenomenon is not well understood and is the subject of current study. The energy expenditure from the hard work of breathing may be one reason. The body simply uses up a lot of energy in the act of breathing. If this is the case, more calories are needed, especially those with high-energy (calorie) value. The highest energy foods contain fats and carbohydrates, but all forms of nutritious food can be converted into the calories required by the body. Thus, one need not force-feed or follow a particularly unusual diet to obtain sufficient calories.

Poor appetite troubles many patients. At times, poor appetite is due to depression, which is a downward change in mood ("the blues") surrounding a serious medical situation. Very often, participation in a comprehensive care or rehabilitation program can reduce or eliminate depression. When depression lifts, appetite improves.

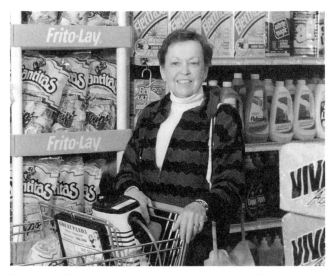

Figure 60. Shopping: Patient doing routine household and grocery shopping. Note the presence of a portable liquid oxygen device in the food basket. This patient is receiving transtracheal oxygen; the tubing is concealed by her clothing.

Many people find shopping and cooking to be great hobbies, as well as nutritional activities. Figure 60 shows a housewife in the grocery story shopping for groceries and household items. Note that her portable liquid oxygen unit is also in her food basket. This patient's use of oxygen is otherwise concealed because it is administered through the transtracheal method and hidden beneath her turtleneck.

Vitamins

It is our opinion that many of the beliefs and clichés regarding vitamins may be wrong. The notion that one gets plenty of vitamins from ordinary food may not apply to the patient with emphysema, or anyone else for that matter, particularly in "older" age groups, i.e., over 50. Although no specific vitamin deficiencies have been identified in patients who consume an appropriate diet, it may well be that extra levels of vitamins could be useful. Many people feel that taking large doses of vitamin C, i.e., up to 1 gram per day, can prevent colds. Some scientific evidence supports this idea. In fact, ascorbic acid (vitamin C) has been under study recently as a possible modifier of bronchospastic reactions within the lungs. Taking citrus fruits daily would provide a good supply of vitamin C. Perhaps taking as much as 500 to 1000 mg of vitamin C daily in addition could be useful for some patients.

Beta carotene, which produces vitamin A and vitamin E, is probably of equal importance. Vitamins A, B, and C are the most commonly used antioxidant vitamins. If COPD is caused by oxidation, perhaps supplemental antioxidant vitamins could be partly protective, but this is a hypothesis that remains to be tested in scientific studies.

The use of one-a-day vitamins of high concentration, such as Stress Caps, is popular among many patients. It is highly unlikely that a vitamin overdose will occur from these products. Thus, we tend to believe that vitamin supplements, including one-a-day multivitamins, are worth a try, particularly for individuals who are suffering weight loss or who are not thriving on an apparently appropriate diet.

Alcohol

Alcohol is actually a food and, like carbohydrates, is metabolized into energy. However, large amounts of alcohol are harmful and can adversely affect the heart, the muscles, and even the lungs. By contrast, small amounts of alcohol are useful and, in fact, may have a health benefit. Three or four ounces of wine, one or two ounces of spirits with or without cocktail mix, or twelve to twenty ounces of beer may well be a useful daily appetite stimulant. As a matter of fact, for those who enjoy beer, a 12-ounce can of regular (not light) beer provides 130 to 170 calories.

Contrary to popular belief, beer does *not* contain much sodium. In fact, it contains less sodium than most water supplies. Thus, beer would be a good beverage for any meal. This is not to say that we condone the excessive use of alcohol. Alcohol dependence can be a serious problem for any patient, particularly one with advanced COPD. We advise the judicious use of alcoholic beverages not only for their pleasure, but for their ability to stimulate appetite. Most importantly, these beverages enhance a meal, and thus encourage an increase in overall caloric intake.

Tranquilizers, Sleeping Pills, and Mood Elevators

As we have already said, many patients with serious degrees of COPD are anxious, depressed, and preoccupied with various bodily functions. This "neurotic triad" has been studied by psychologists and psychiatrists. We have done a number of evaluations in our own patients and know that these observations are correct. We also have found that participation in a patient-education program and the additional approaches to rehabilitation discussed in this book are extremely powerful tools in overcoming these reactions to illness. These reactions are a result of— and *not* the cause of—the disease. Their solution rarely requires deep psychotherapy; usually the patient's personal physician can treat these symptoms effectively.

Drug therapy for these "nervous states" might be useful, but excessive use of tranquilizers or sedatives can be quite harmful. Any use of sedatives, tranquilizers, or mood-elevating drugs should be undertaken only under the strict prescription of your personal physician.

Having offered this caution, we would like to state clearly that the judicious use of certain drugs that enhance relaxation and sleep and elevate mood can be useful. First, antidepressants such as Elavil® (amitriptyline), Tofranil® (imipramine), Haldol® (haloperidol), and newer drugs such as Prozac® (fluoxetine), can help to combat the type of depression that leads to agitation and insomnia. Generally, small doses are used. Often the doctor prescribes these drugs for use at bedtime because the control of an agitated depression may lead to marked sleepiness. When such drugs promote normal nighttime sleep, considerable benefit is gained.

In addition, the judicious use of small amounts of tranquilizers, such as Librium® (chlordiazepoxide) or Valium® (diazepam), can be helpful when taken at bedtime. These drugs are feared by physicians because they can decrease the drive to breathe by suppressing the control center for breathing within the brain. However, small doses of Valium (2 mg) or Librium (2 or 5 mg) are well tolerated in many individuals without causing respiratory depression.

These same drugs can be used as "sleeping pills." Small amounts of older short-acting barbiturates can also be used for this purpose, starting with a small dose and building up gradually as necessary. However, it is best not to rely on sleeping pills every evening.

Personal Hygiene

Bathing, shampooing, and dressing are difficult for many patients with COPD because of the increased energy and breathing that these activities require. Generally, showering is most efficient, since it allows the patient to both shampoo and shower in a short period of time. Some people feel choked from the high humidity of the shower or bath. Also, just getting in and out of the shower, if it requires stepping into the bathtub, may be difficult. The act of washing the body, too, may cause shortness of breath. When this occurs, the spouse or a friend should help with bathing. In addition, it may be useful to use a wooden stool to sit on while showering. The stool helps one to get in and out of the bathtub as well. Also, simply coordinating one's breathing pattern while getting in and out of the bathtub or shower can help.

Some patients look upon bathing as agony because of the shortness of breath it causes. This attitude is sad and can generally be overcome with some counseling and the development of coping mechanisms against shortness of breath. When things still remain difficult, reducing the frequency of bathing is certainly appropriate. Few people need a daily bath. Simply washing personal areas with a washcloth is sufficient in most situations, and shampoos in the sink are entirely satisfactory. Use a hair dryer on your head and on your bottom, too. It works both ways!

Suggestions from a Patient

The following is a letter we received from Mrs. Carole L. Wolfe after she read the first edition:

Sometimes it's hard to feel feminine with this disease. I've been married 26 years and had always felt good about myself but have had to resort to some tricks to pull myself back up:

- *Keep fingernails and toenails filed, cut, and painted. Get creative. One doesn't need to go to a professional manicurist for the "latest" in nail fashion . . . "go for it," get artificial ones if you need to.*

- *Why buy or wear plain white unmentionables when you can wear lacy whatevers, or colored matching you-know-whats. Everything needs replacing sometime . . . replace with something that would make your mother blush. If you can't* replace—*then get out the Rit Dye and dye it a color that would make Tina Turner blush; see the next item if you don't know who "Tina Turner" is . . .*

- Read *not just about your disease, but about what is happening all over the world and about you and "Ole." Watch MTV. (Never mind, maybe I've gone tooooo far . . .)*

- *Wear* bright *colors . . . even if you don't want to. Especially if you don't want to. If it doesn't cheer you up, it will someone else and* they *will cheer you up.*

- *If you have a water container by your bed that came from the hospital, pick it up and throw it! Get out something that your grandmother used at her tea parties. The more breakable and delicate the better! Don't be practical about something you look at and use so often . . . The same applies to:*

- Kleenex—*either get a pretty holder or at the very least, decorated box.*

- *Put your pills in a basket trimmed in lace. (Do it yourself; all you have to do is* glue—*real easy after you've gotten the basket and lace).*

- *The bedroom doesn't need to look like a hospital, and changes can be made without costing a lot.*

- *I made a quilted cover for my portable oxygen tank—I wasn't trying to hide the* fact . . .*just the* ugly *tank. Most medical equipment is painted a drab color, and if it is possible, paint it or sew cushions, etc.*
- *Wear two things frivolous. One that others can see . . . and something only a (chosen) few know about . . . In my case, I forgot about the medical profession and jumped a foot when asked, "What's that?" by a nurse. (Doesn't* everyone *wear a tiny linked chain around their [big] waist?) At least, I didn't get the tattoo (just kidding)! It (the chain) also serves a* medical *purpose: It will* break *if I eat too much!!!*

These things may seem a little extreme . . . Why not?

A "fun" thing I'm "working on" now is going with a particular friend to every restaurant in town (Ridgecrest is a fairly small town—about 26,000) for breakfast. My husband doesn't like to eat out that much and my friend loves breakfast—I don't always feel so good in the morning, etc. so I'm sure we'll always have new choices of where to go, etc.

Also the post office has service by mail (for stamps) and most banks have some sort of services for the disabled. Also, apply for disabled parking plates if you are eligible . . . If you only have so much energy, take advantage of services and use the extra time or energy in a way that will be more rewarding to you.

Dressing

A number of helpful hints assist the emphysema patient in dressing. These individuals have their greatest problems while bending over to put on or tie shoes; while pulling sweaters, blouses, and other garments over the head; and while pulling up pants and trousers. In general, it is best to coordinate the breathing sequence during dressing. Additional helpful hints include a long-handled shoe horn for putting on shoes, suspenders rather than belts (which also helps remove any feeling of constriction around the abdomen), and choosing blouses and sweaters that button rather than pull over. These suggestions may seem simple, but many patients do not think of them.

We are well aware that we have not considered every possible activity of daily living. This chapter is simply intended to touch on common daily activities that may at times be difficult for the patient with COPD. We always need additional suggestions and hints for our patients, so if you have some new ideas please let us know. Notice that in Chapter 17 we specifically ask you to make this contribution to those who suffer from COPD.

Suggested Reading

Non-scientific:

1. Dewey J: Of Life and Breath. New York, Warner Books, 1986.

2. Shayevitz MB and Shayevitz BR: Living Well with Emphysema and Bronchitis. New York, Doubleday, 1985.

3. "Letters From Tom." Available from my office at Presbyterian/St. Luke's Medical Center, 1719 E. 19th Avenue, Denver, Colorado 80218. FAX No. (303) 832–5137.

CHAPTER FIFTEEN

HOME CARE

The concept of home care is rapidly becoming reestablished for patients with any form of chronic illness. Of course, there is nothing new about home care. In the pre-high-technology era, the management of patients with chronic illnesses of all sorts focused on the home. Family members and, on some occasions, visiting nurses helped provide comfort and the limited drug therapy that was then available. In fact, a few patients requiring continuous mechanical ventilation in the polio era lived at home, usually with the help of unique family members, and more rarely, private duty nurses. Some patients continue to receive this kind of life support in the home.

Three major factors have contributed to the resurgence of home care for many patients with COPD. The first of these was the availability of home oxygen, which first became popular in the mid–1970s. Today, 800,000 to 1,000,000 individuals are receiving oxygen at home. The expanded oxygen supply industry has helped make this possible. New advances in oxygen therapy technology and its use in selected patients with COPD are discussed in Chapter 6. Requirements for prescribing oxygen under Health Care Financing Administration regulations are also covered in the Oxygen Consensus Conference references at the end of Chapter 6.

The second major factor that is shifting the emphasis of care back to the home is the use of diagnosis related groups (DRGs) for Medicare and Medicaid reimbursements. DRGs have standardized the reimbursements hospitals receive for specific diagnoses. For example, if a patient is admitted for COPD, DRG #88, the hospital is reimbursed for only 6.6 days of hospitalization. Since this is the maximum payment a hospital will receive, there is a strong incentive for patients to be discharged quickly, before the 6.6-day limit is reached.

There are advantages to home care which are pretty obvious. The comfort of living in one's own surroundings is probably the most important reason for the increased emphasis on home care. There is no particular reason why intravenous antibiotics and other drugs, in addition to oxygen, cannot be given at home. Also, nutritional support beyond ordinary food can also be prescribed in the home setting.

Since it is obviously far less expensive to provide these services in the home (compared to the hospital), a proliferation of private home health services is now occurring. When home health care services are appropriately utilized, their costs can be reimbursed by third party payers. Reimbursement is not presently limited by the DRG concept but, of course, that is always possible in the future.

Currently, a movement toward home mechanical ventilation is again occurring. We don't expect that many patients with COPD will choose to live the last part of their lifetime supported by a mechanical ventilator at home. But in certain instances where the quality of life is good, this is one option. An increasing number of reliable and practical mechanical ventilators, including some that can be powered by batteries, are now available.

It is likely that short periods of mechanical ventilation in the home could be used to rest respiratory muscles fatigued by the work of breathing in states of advanced COPD. There are presently several studies under way which will determine whether or not sleeping on a mechanical ventilator for 8 to 10 hours might afford the necessary relief to allow for recovery. In these instances, mechanical ventilation could be applied by a mask attached to the face or nose. Another method is "negative pressure ventilation;" here, something like a shell or body-wrap encases the patient. The respirator then intermittently creates a vacuum around the patient's chest, allowing for the inflow of air during the inspiratory phase of breathing. This technique is akin to the use of the old-fashioned "iron lung" of the polio era. Indeed, the iron lung is still used in a few areas of the world.

The decision to employ mechanical ventilation, of course, is a complex one to be made by physician and patient, in the context of the family support system available. Economics will be another consideration. It is the purpose of this chapter only to introduce the fact that:

1. The technology exists;
2. The likelihood of benefit in selected patients is real;
3. Home health care services are expanding to meet an anticipated need for more and more patients to receive either short or prolonged periods of mechanical ventilation in the home setting.

Thus, home care is rapidly returning to the American health care system. It is our prediction that home care will become increasingly more popular as a means of providing cost-effective care for COPD patients whose quality of life remains good in spite of the necessity of mechanical ventilation. Whether or not large numbers of patients will benefit as they have from home oxygen therapy remains to be seen. Of course, all of the patient's care requirements (drugs, nutrition, physical therapy, etc.) must be integrated into a successful home care program.

Suggested Reading

Publications in the medical literature:

Home Health Care, by the Health and Public Policy Committee of the American College of Physicians—Ann Intern Med 1986;105:454–460.

Medical News and Perspectives

Caring for Elderly: Challenge for now and 21st century medicine. JAMA 1986;255:3057–3058.

Editorials:

Korin MJ: Home care—who cares? N Engl J Med 1986;314: 917–920.

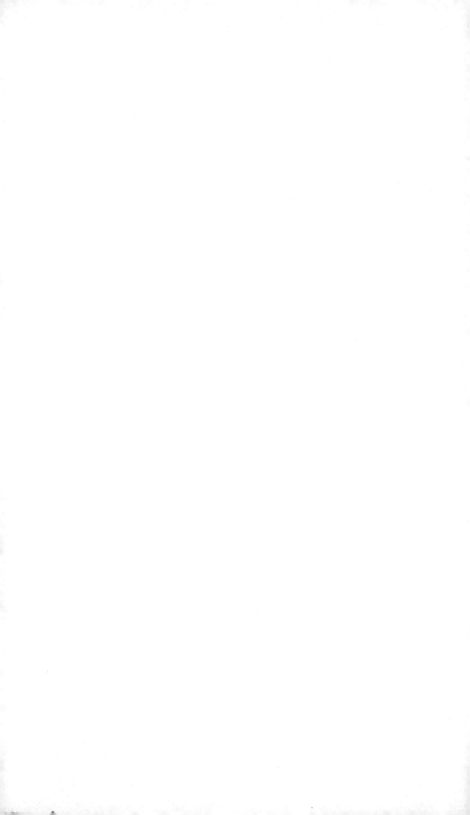

CHAPTER SIXTEEN

THE FUTURE

Research and The Final Solution to COPD

We are enthusiastic about the current prospects for finding the final solution to the COPD problem within this century. After all, we know the greatest risk factors for this disease, which relate primarily to smoking and family history. We know that the disease process covers 20 to 40 years and is slowly progressive. COPD comes on inexorably, although the patient *may not be aware* of emerging emphysema or chronic bronchitis. Most likely, the patient simply denies early symptoms that could be important signs of disease. If an individual were to respond to these signals, early identification and intervention would be possible.

Of great importance is the fact that we have an excellent tool for identifying all stages of COPD. This tool is the simple airflow test, the FEV_1 performed with a spirometer (see Chapter 3). It is time to put a spirometer (just like a blood pressure cuff) in all physicians' offices for early detection of disease.

There is no question that the early identification of COPD could change its course dramatically. Abnormalities detected early on might convince patients to modify their smoking behavior, perhaps change their place of residence, or even switch occupations if appropriate as an investment in lung health and in their future health. We now know the risks of COPD, understand the course of the disease, and have an excellent tool for identification, the spirometer. We have an excellent intervention (smoking cessation). In addition, we believe that the early use of bronchodilators could help stem the progress of disease. With only the knowledge we have today, we could dramatically reduce the impact of this disease immediately.

The Lung Division of the National Heart, Lung and Blood Institute, a major component of the National Institutes of Health, along with ten selected medical centers, has just reported on a nationwide program for early identification and intervention in COPD. We are proud of this effort, which was initiated during the author's (TLP's) term as President of the American College of Chest Physicians, with the strong support of the co-author (LMN). The effects and clinical and social values of early identification and intervention in the early stages of COPD were evaluated in this multicenter, controlled clinical trial. The intervention included smoking cessation and the use of simple and safe bronchodilator drugs.

The results of this study, presented at the 1994 annual meeting of the American Thoracic Society, are truly exciting. With special efforts, nearly 40% of patients with early stages of COPD were finally assisted in a successful smoking cessation effort. The rate of lung function degeneration was better in people who stopped smoking compared with those who continued. The bronchodilator ipratropium bromide (Atrovent) increased lung function. When patients were tested without Atrovent, there appeared to be no change in the course of lung function reduction. The important point was that Atrovent continued to work as a bronchodilator as long as it was used in this 5-year study.

The best method for implementing a new nationwide program to treat COPD early remains to be determined. Certainly it will require that the media, the medical, nursing, and respiratory therapy professions, and society be informed on the subject. Industry, unions, and government must also show interest in bringing about such a program. Since the early identification of COPD is in the best interests of everyone, socially as well as economically, we feel that a nationwide early identification program will be developed and effectively implemented in the not-too-distant future.

It is likely that the new interest in health through fitness, along with the emergence of health concerns about the environment and the work place, can motivate change. Most important of all, of course, is personal motivation and control over one's personal environment. Attention to this fact is more important than all other efforts to improve lung health.

As we write this third edition, scientists continue to make major breakthroughs in understanding how tobacco smoke damages the lung. The protective material, alpha–1-antitrypsin or alpha antitrypsin (AAT), which combats enzymatic damage of the lung, is fortunately present in normal amounts in most of our citizens. Only a few persons have the genetic deficiency state that makes them vulnerable to lung damage. Cigarette smoke, however, can destroy AAT even in those born with normal amounts of it. Finding ways to protect AAT so it can combat enzymatic damage would be a major breakthrough in treatment. Drugs that appear to accomplish this feat are already under study. It is possible, in fact, to increase levels of AAT via the use of some drugs or even to replace it, much like giving gamma globulin shots (see Chapter 5). None of these approaches for augmenting AAT or its protective function is yet practical and so is not available to patients. Nonetheless, this research is a step in the right direction and will ultimately lead to a basic biological treatment for a special form of emphysema within the spectrum of COPD.

Therefore, with a concerted nationwide effort to identify and intervene early with appropriate behavioral modifications for those at risk, and with a new biological approach made available through unique drug interventions, we can look forward to major reductions in the impact of COPD in the years to come.

How great it would be for our country to avoid the $80 billion drain caused by COPD. How much better for families not to have to suffer the consequences of COPD in a loved one. How much better for the patient to enjoy life fully through an unrestricted ability to live and breathe!

Your Personal Future

• **What is Your Future Now?** Questions about the future, of course, are on the mind of anyone with any form of illness, particularly chronic illness that by its very nature is progressive. Obviously, making absolute predictions about anyone's future is impossible. Yet we know so much about the course of COPD that some reasonable predictions can be made. These are always of interest to patients and their families.

• **How Long Will You Live?** This, of course, depends on many factors. Most significant are the age at which emphysema is diagnosed and the degree of lung function impairment present. For example, it was pointed out in Chapter 3 that a simple flow test, the FEV_1, is an important predictor of outcome. The use of FEV_1 in emphysema is much like that of the diastolic blood pressure in predicting outcome from hypertension. When one declines to an FEV_1 of 1 liter, significant functional impairment is present. Even when the FEV_1 is 1.5 to 2 liters, the patient almost always has shortness of breath upon exertion. However, the rate of decline is also very important. For example, an FEV_1 of 2 liters at age 40 in an average-sized man means he has lost approximately half of his lung function over a short span of time. If the FEV_1 is 2 liters at age 60, the same degree of impairment obviously has taken much longer to occur, and so the progression of disease has been much slower. If the FEV_1 is 2 liters at age 80, lung function is probably normal.

Take this a step further and consider an FEV_1 of 1 liter at age 40, age 60, and age 80. People with an FEV_1 of 1 liter at age 60 have approximately a 50% chance of living 5 years or more. Those with an FEV_1 of 1 liter at age 80 have already lived a normal lifespan; since it has taken 80 years to get down to an FEV_1 of 1 liter, the rate of deterioration has been extremely slow. This patient probably will live quite a few more years without much progression of disease. At the other extreme, patients with an FEV_1 of 1 liter at age 40 have the most rapidly progressive disease, often due to an AAT deficiency.

If there is a major degree of reversibility in the FEV_1, i.e., improvement following the use of bronchodilator drugs or corticosteroids, the prognostic estimate can be modified upward. If, by contrast, there is no reversibility, the prognosis is not as good. Finally, the rate of change over time, i.e., the slope of deterioration, gives the physician the best indication about a long-term prognosis. Thus, serial lung-function tests done annually or every other year will help to plot the course of COPD and help estimate long-term survival.

• **How Well Will You Live?** To many, this question is much more important than the previous one. After all, it is the quality of life that makes it worthwhile. The ability to enjoy, to feel the fruits of productivity, to relish the satisfaction of one's contributions to others, and to feel contentment over one's own accomplishments create peace and tranquility in the minds of most persons. Yet, in the face of chronic illness, one must sometimes *work* at enjoyment. Patients must learn to plan on fun and zestful living, no matter what degree of respiratory impairment may be present. This notion is so important that the last chapter of this book is an appeal: *Remember to Live!*

• **What Next?** What is the final outcome of COPD? What will finally happen to you? You have answered this question for yourself many times. You and everyone else will finally die. Why is it so difficult to consider this concept? The answer is that our society is not well prepared for the certainty of death, although we all know it is inevitable. We deny this possibility so many times or perhaps, more accurately, postpone considering its eventuality. The denial of death, after all, is not a bad defense mechanism against anxieties about death. On the other hand, many believe that a positive assessment of the situation and an acceptance of reality through necessary emotional adjustments are far better coping mechanisms. With this in mind, we often have a serious conversation with our patients regarding the future. We call this "the talk."

In "the talk," we discuss the future, the death transition, and how it will occur. When we can have "the talk" under the right circumstances and with appropriate timing, it turns into a magnificent experience for patients, for families, and for us. Powerful human interaction occurs during this session, and frank and honest detailed discussion about the mechanism and phenomenon of death takes place. We emphasize that most patients simply slip into a semi-stuporous state that is quite pleasant. This stuporous state is caused by the buildup of carbon dioxide, a narcotizing agent. Individuals may slip in and out of this state and, in fact, awaken refreshed through mechanisms that are not entirely known. Very likely, the complete relaxation that occurs from carbon dioxide buildup offers rest for both mind and body, thereby leading to a state of temporary recovery. These episodes of recovery may recur over some months or even years.

Death itself is likened to a long sleep. After all, people look forward to sleep for rest, and a long sleep is certain to be especially restful. This concept is very acceptable to patients and families. Yet we never have this discussion without considerable emotion. Often the patients cry, the families cry, and *we* cry, signifying the emotional impact of saying good-bye. After this event, there is an amazing period of tranquility. We call this a détente, i.e., a détente with death in its real or perceived meaning.

Many patients have lived months or even a few years after this discussion and counseling session. Actually, it does no harm to deal somewhat prematurely with the issues concerning death because, after all, both the patient and the family have concerns, anxieties, and fantasies that should be addressed. Dealing with reality and developing confidence based on guidance are helpful and may prevent some of the concerns that preoccupy the patient and his or her family. This preoccupation can totally interfere with the enjoyment and living that remain.

Additional counseling may be necessary as time goes on to reinforce the basic concept that death is an entirely natural event, guaranteed from the moment of conception.

Our society's fear of death is a matter of concern for all of us and a subject of study for anthropologists, sociologists, and theologians. No one is promised immortality. Even in health, our biological clock is roughly preset for the length of life. Consider the fact that no more people are living to age 80, 90, or 100 today than they were at the beginning of this century.

All organ system functions deteriorate naturally as we age. Even simple connective tissue cells, called fibroblasts, grown in laboratory cultures can only multiply approximately 50 times. Then, although nutritional, environmental, and growth factors do not change, these cells reveal their mortality and fail to survive. There appears to be such a time limit for all normal biological cells.

By contrast, abnormal cells, i.e., cancer cells, can be kept in tissue culture in perpetuity, thus suggesting their immortality. It is interesting to consider that malignant cells are potentially immortal and, in fact, cause death of the normal body when regulatory mechanisms, i.e., intrinsic control of the cancer process, fail. Thus, this control process not only limits the length of our life, but protects it along the way.

Our job as medical professionals is to *prevent premature morbidity and mortality*. We are now able through the advances of medicine to live closer and closer to the length of time allotted by our biological control systems. The length of the lives of patients with COPD has been dramatically increased by successful treatment in intensive-care units where medical emergencies, such as acute respiratory failure, are effectively managed.

Beyond this obvious advance are the improved length and quality of life that result from pulmonary rehabilitation programs, including home oxygen. The added length of life can be many years, even up to a decade or more. Hopefully, the time "bought" by forestalling premature morbidity and mortality is useful and pleasant, but it is not intended to last forever.

Remember that birth, life, and death are natural phenomena. Try to die of "nothing serious."

We are mindful of Psalm 90, which states, "The years of our life shall be three score and ten years, but if by reason of strength, they may be four score years." Hopefully, current strategies intended to enhance the life and happiness of patients with COPD can help them live this long. In fact, most patients with emphysema are now reaching their late 60s and 70s, and some live well into old age.

The Psalm continues, " . . . and then the spirit takes wings and flies away."

CHAPTER SEVENTEEN

REMEMBER TO LIVE!

The late Alvan Barach of New York, one of the true pioneers in the care of patients with emphysema—and a world class humanist—often spoke on the subject, "Remember to Live." His message was an admonition to all that, in spite of difficulties and impediments, we must remember to live. He wrote the following poem, which was published in the *Journal of the American Medical Association* (August 23, 1971):

> *Doctor, Be Careful of Being Careful*
>
> *Doctors who budget pleasure with a stoic air*
> *Preach pastoral living in their office lair,*
> *Loathe to reveal dame Nature's laws,*
> *To Don'ts and to Denials give much applause,*
> *And to the "id" too little trust!*
> *Since man for long will not eat dust,*
> *Ripe physicians, wary of abstemious hours*
> *And of idle and hoarded powers*
> *Stress engagement and the ploys of pleasure*
> *Expanded living, experience in full measure.*

We should gear ourselves for pleasant and fulfilling living in spite of all impairments, whether they be inadequate financial resources or poor physical health. We must capitalize on our resources and minimize our restrictions, whatever they may be. In short, we must reprogram ourselves for pleasant living on a *prospective basis*, now and for the rest of our lives. After all, "Today is the first day of the rest of your life." This concept is depicted in Figure 61, a drawing that suggests a new awakening of interest in living.

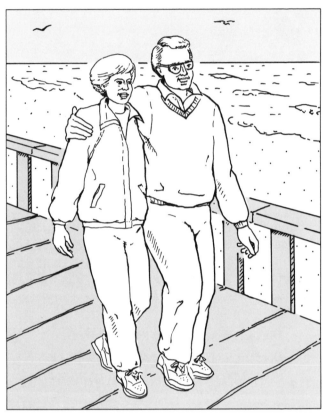

Figure 61. Enjoy Life: This figure symbolizes a new awakening and interest in life through learning to cope with COPD and increasing one's horizons through expanded activities of daily living. Consider yourself in this picture.

Let us just for a moment differentiate between disease and illness. A disease is an impairment of an organ system in terms of its structure or function. An illness is the total impact of that impairment on the integrated functioning of the person. Illness deals with failure to adapt and with impairment, or the perception of impairment, that interferes with daily living. Thus, one can have a significant disease without illness or considerable illness with trivial disease. The illness aspect of a disease, however, deals with the whole psychosocial and cultural composition of the individual. It is sometimes taught that this response to disease is preset or pre-determined. We don't believe this notion, since we have seen many people adjust quite successfully to great impairments. Whether or not this adaptation is acquired or is present all along makes absolutely no difference, since the necessary adjustment to the disease occurs in either case. Hopefully the advice and philosophy presented in this chapter will either reawaken adaptive capabilities or offer new guidelines for acquiring these highly useful resources.

One of Dr. Barach's favorite quotations was that of Thomas Carlyle: "The tragedy in men's lives is not what they suffer, but what they miss" (see Chapter 10). We have always thought that this quotation is applicable to our patients and to ourselves. True, our patients may suffer from the impairments of COPD, but all too often this "suffering" is blown totally out of proportion and dominates their lives, causing them to miss much of what lies ahead. Philosophers

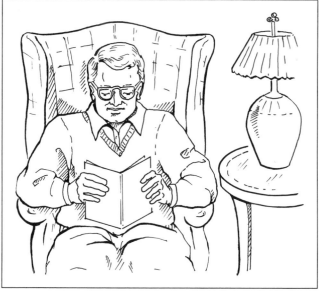

Figure 62. Read and Learn: Learn about enjoying life with COPD through reading books such as this and others. You should become an expert in your own health care.

have obviously pondered this point, e.g., Tennyson, "As if to breathe were life."

It should be apparent to all who have read this book that we intend to give the individual new resources and guidelines for enjoying life. We hope that the basic descriptive chapters on disease processes, the course and prognosis of disease, and methods of care will help to provide the educational background for coping with COPD and enjoying life. We have always felt that a clear understanding of the disease, the goals of management, and individual responses to the stresses of illness are valuable scaffolding for building a sound and satisfying future. This is why we wrote this book (Figure 62); we intend that patients and their families study it carefully, but we also wrote it for health workers (see Preface). Naturally, we cannot restructure the educational, socioeconomic, and cultural background of every person who reads this book. We simply hope that reviewing and making an inventory of one's own resources will be helpful. This process can hopefully reawaken adaptive strengths and stimulate the acquisition of new approaches to life, which must now be done on a prospective basis.

Like Barach, we are particularly fond of a quotation from the late Cardinal Newman: "A man would do nothing if he waited until he could do it so well that no one would find fault with what he has done."

The following paragraphs present a few ideas to help you to organize your own thinking and to pursue life in a more useful way.

Don't Be Afraid to Take Medicine

Many patients are reluctant to follow their doctor's advice because they fear the toxicities of medicine. Alternatively, they feel that postponing these medications will make them more valuable in the future when they are "really needed." This reluctance is unfounded and inappropriate.

There is no known serious long-term toxicity from bronchodilators and antibiotics given in usual doses. By contrast, there are long-term toxicities from corticosteroids, e.g., prednisone and prednisolone. These long-term side effects include a weakening of bones (osteoporosis), accelerated cataract formation, and thinning of skin in some people. These facts were discussed in Chapter 5. But if corticosteroids can be used to improve airflow and restore the functioning of the individual, increased activity may itself prevent osteoporosis. If a drug is effective and produces true measured benefit, we believe it is important to use it for the value it offers *now*, rather than discarding it for fear of future complications that may be entirely unfounded. Wouldn't it be a pity to realize the tremendous value of corticosteroids 10 years later than was necessary? Of course, it must be your physician's decision to prescribe these medications. The use of all medical therapy, we feel, should be a contract between the enlightened patient and an experienced physician whose goal is the same: The happy functioning of the patient for the longest possible time.

Don't Postpone Pleasure

It never ceases to amaze us when people who have clear-cut plans for future enjoyment postpone them inappropriately and indefinitely. Although we remain conservative in philosophy, it is not conservative, but rather reactionary, to postpone travel, adventure, or experimentation with new life situations for no real reason. Fears about the economy, future wars, nuclear holocaust, or other environmental or personal catastrophes should not govern your activity. How can we promote this idea in our patients?

Perhaps it is best dealt with by you, the individual. How many times have you feared doing something (making an investment, taking a trip, or trying something different) and have not done it, only to find out that your fear was unfounded? In other words, your fears just didn't come true.

Ask yourself another question. How many times have you made a really disastrous mistake? Of course, we have all made mistakes, but we overcome them, reorient ourselves, and adventure once again. We would like to encourage and promote this attitude toward life. Certainly, prudent planning for the future, both economically and in relation to one's health, is a necessity. But again, abandoning an opportunity out of unreasonable fear is usually inappropriate.

Again we refer to our friend, the late Alvan Barach of New York, by quoting an article he wrote for physicians in the journal *Geriatrics* more than 25 years ago.

STORAGE OF PLEASURES:
THE PHYSICIAN'S ROLE
Alvan L. Barach, M.D.

A storage of pleasure may be vital help when there is a run of bad luck. Misfortune is at times inevitable, but the misery of illness is frequently overcast with what we are forced to miss as a result. In fact, the lack of life's customary activities has resulted in more suffering for some people than the symptoms of a disease itself. How high a price must a patient pay for the discontents of civilization—the omission of pleasurable activities?

The charismatic influence of the physician is such that he may do something to lessen that price or, unhappily, he may curb the solaces that some patients need. Consider the individual who is breathless on exertion, since unusual publicity has been accorded recently to the remarkable increase in incidence of pulmonary emphysema. Although more skillful testing of the syndrome probably accounts for its increased recognition, there has been an unusual stimulation of research, and cigarette smoking has been indicated as a cause or at least an aggravator of the condition. Thus, one of the man's oldest solaces has been taken away.

Since the prohibitionist has [long ago—editor] folded his tents, alcohol in moderation generally is allowed. However, some doctors are more strict than others. A patient with pulmonary emphysema was presented at a medical staff meeting and, during the recital of his history, the physician frowned as he said, 'This man drinks a pint of whiskey every day.' A more liberal-minded colleague sought to put the patient at ease by remarking, 'My patients spill that much.' I once suggested that an alcoholic is a man who drinks more than his own doctor; this general thesis seems to be applicable to enjoyments other than alcohol.

Of the remaining solaces man has heralded, women and song appear to be too ticklish to discuss in this brief exposition. There are, of course, less spectacular enjoyments, such as the theater, movies, parties, athletics, games, and travel, as well as the more pastoral recreations of reading and writing. Many out-of-door activities require physical health of a degree.

Unfortunately, the adage 'conserve the energies of older people' has influenced some physicians (often those who chose medicine as a last-minute switch from the ministry) to urge their patients to stay at home. Dyspnea is relieved at rest for most patients with emphysema. But what is the cost in terms of the life that has been missed? Not all people can be appeased by medication and its allied pursuits.

I suggest that we prepare these older people for a rainy day by encouraging them to store pleasures. A pleasure once had cannot be taken away. Let them pile up a number of diversions and put them away in the bank of memory as a reserve to draw upon for the days when life seems especially thin. For, if a patient is living on a small margin of experienced enjoyments, a run on his bank may result in bankruptcy of the most vicious kind—depression, anxiety, and the hysterical symptom of hyperventilation, as he cries, 'Air, air!'

Suppose the patient needs supportive oxygen to perform the activities that he longs for. So what? Supply it as one supplies insulin for the diabetic. I do not propose the inhalation of oxygen just to enable patients to walk across the room without dyspnea, or to climb stairs, or to use a treadmill. Not at all! It is to make possible the same activities that men and women without dyspnea are fond of.

Our mission as physicians is not simply to prolong life, but to contribute to making it absorbing, too. It is common to say that one only lives once, but some people don't even do that. Let's help, not hinder that experience, if indeed it should turn out to be, for once.

This is an age when the doctor employs so many don'ts and preaches giving up so many things—milk and eggs, salt and cream, alcohol and tobacco—even emigration from the city the patient loves to less polluted wide-open spaces where he has little to interest him. In an age like this, it seems timely to present the positive side. Let's ask the patient what he has missed through his illness or what he may now be missing. Some patients say that it costs so much to go to dinner and the theater. The physician can reply, 'It's cheaper than seeing me.'

Reprint of guest editorial, Geriatrics, *July 1967*

Don't Give Up Your Job or Your House Too Soon

Many people feel that if they simplify their lives, things will go better. This often leads to premature retirement or moving into a more "convenient" residence. There are some real problems with these decisions.

A person's vocation is important not only because of financial rewards, but for the feelings of personal accomplishment which are often not considered when one decides to retire prematurely. Almost everyone pursues their employment from a creative point of view. Giving this up has its "down side." It is highly likely that people give up both pleasure and adaptation to life by premature retirement (see Chapter 9). By all means, the final decision for retirement rests with the individual, but deep and thoughtful consideration, with counseling from physicians and other health workers about the impact of retirement, should be a high priority.

Giving up one's home to move to an apartment or condominium also has its disadvantages. When one does this one gives up part of one's usual environment, which includes items of memory, space, a yard for interaction with nature, and opportunities for recreation (see Chapter 10). Is it really wise to give up a major part of your present environment? Is it time to reduce your space? These are serious questions. Certainly, if the energy requirements of living in the home environment exceed the capability of the individual, then simplifying one's life in the interests of "efficiency" does make sense. Our only concern is for the patient who takes this step prematurely. We feel particularly concerned about elderly people who hasten to enter retirement homes prematurely, again hoping for simplicity, peace, and tranquility. This move often represents a significant lifestyle change with adverse social consequences. At times, the interaction with elderly and often considerably impaired and disabled persons can be positive. All too often it is negative, however, and the individual becomes involved in the illnesses of others on top of their own. Thus, again, we must give careful consideration to our place of residence at retirement and in older age.

Continue to Grow and to Improve Yourself

"A man is not old as long as he is seeking something."

JEAN RUSTAND

It seems to us that since we have been growing in some capacity all of our lives, we should continue to grow forever or at least until the end of life. Many highly productive people well into their 80s, 90s, and beyond have proven this ability.

Why can some people continue to grow and others not? Naturally, we do not have a simple answer to this big question. We suspect, however, that it is a matter of attitude and dedication to the growth process itself. Those who have continued to grow throughout their lives could have become stagnant along the way, but for some reason they didn't. These individuals probably enjoyed the feeling of growth and accomplishment and were wise enough to reject the admonitions so often associated with old age that only lead to unhappiness. These attitudes are ingrained in our daily conversation. How many times have you heard, "Dad, don't be so foolish to climb the ladder (paint the house; shingle the roof)," or "Mom, why don't you act your age?", or "Hello, you old fool!", or "You dirty old man!"? Why do people give up so much with the passage of time?

"But," you may say, "what can I do with my problem?" This, of course, depends on your interests and resources. Certainly you can read different things, talk to new people, develop new ideas, and take on new challenges. We are convinced that this is possible in view of our work with so many disabled people in all age groups with many different diseases. Here we are speaking particularly of patients with various paralytic disorders, such as those with polio of years past, young people with muscular dystrophy, children and young adults with cystic fibrosis, and people with other serious impairments. It would take more pages than this entire book to recount all the accomplishments made by people with serious impairments. Somehow, the human spirit possesses an ability to adapt and grow, which we believe can be awakened and kindled for the pursuit of happiness at any time in life.

We end this book with a request from you, the reader, for ideas of your own. Now, we have you exactly where we want you. We are asking you to be creative in your own mind and to think of something new for our benefit, as well as for yours. We want your ideas so that we can better understand COPD from a patient's point of view. We want to learn more about how people cope with this disease, even though we have been studying this topic for more than 30 years.

Write us a letter with specific ideas and suggestions. By doing so you can participate in the interactive process of advancing knowledge through communication. If you will only let us know your ideas, you will be assisting us in writing the next message for our patients, and our own knowledge and ability will be enhanced. If you haven't noticed it already, we, like you, are trying to adapt, learn, and grow.

Quite frankly, we have enjoyed the process of creating this third edition. Indeed, many have responded with their reactions to the first two editions and several have offered constructive criticism and advice, which have been embodied in these pages. We thank all who have responded.

"Were it offered to my choice, I should have no objection to a repetition of the same life from its beginning, only asking the advantages authors have in a second edition to correct some of the faults in the first."

BENJAMIN FRANKLIN

GLOSSARY OF TERMS[1]

aerosol: A fine particle spray. Inhaled bronchodilators are aerosols.

aerosolize: The act of nebulizing medications for inhalation into the lungs.

air hunger: The sensation of insufficient oxygen or difficult breathing.

air pollution: This term refers to grossly polluted air in our cities. Air pollution consists of hydrocarbons from automobile exhaust resulting in oxides of nitrogen and ozone sulfur and carbon monoxide.

Whereas the dusty air of the plains is impressive, the inhalation of this ground dust is probably not harmful to the lungs. People in various industries are exposed to various dusts that can cause harm. Most individuals who feel irritation while at work are actually heavy smokers and fail to realize that their cough and expectoration are coming from smoking tobacco or other materials. Smoking and industrial air pollution are additive hazards.

allergy: Abnormal reaction to a stimulus called an allergen. Allergy refers to the abnormal response of the airways to inhaled stimuli, such as pollen, or to consumed items, such as foods, that may cause unusual airway reaction leading to bronchospasm.

---

[1]Terms of general interest to the reader of this book. Not all these terms are used in the book itself. The list is not complete and does not include all terms of interest to our readers. When necessary, please refer to a general or medical dictionary.

alpha antitrypsin (AAT): Also called alpha antiprotein-
ase (AAP). This is a protective material in our lungs. It
is produced in the liver and transported to the lungs to
help combat inflammation. Deficiency states can occur
as the result of hereditary defects (rare) or can be
acquired by tobacco smoking (common).

alveoli: Folded sac-like structures at the end of the conducting airways in which the exchange of oxygen and
carbon dioxide takes place. (See Figures 1 and 3, Chapter 1.)

antibiotic: A drug that kills or inhibits bacteria. Antibiotics are effective in combating deep chest infections in
which bacterial invasions are almost always present.
It should be stressed that antibiotics do not prevent the
common cold and will not stop a cold that has developed.
These drugs are simply effective against the bacterial
invaders that follow the original cold virus.

antidepressant: A drug used to treat depression, e.g.,
Elavil (amitriptyline), Haldol (haloperidol).

autonomic nerves: Nerves that control organ functions,
i.e., visceral nerves. Nervous impulses may alter various organ functions, including the functions of the
lungs.

bacteria: Infectious organisms that may cause bronchitis
or pneumonia.

basal state: State of minimum metabolism in which oxygen requirements are lowest.

black pigment: The material that gives damaged human
lungs the black and sooty appearance. The exact iden-
tity of the pigment has never been determined, but it
is related to cigarette smoking and to urban living. It
is always found in patients with emphysema or chronic
bronchitis.

blebs and bullae: Localized destroyed portions of the
lungs that may occupy large portions of the thorax and
occasionally compress otherwise useful lungs.

blood gas determinations: The direct measurement of oxygen and carbon dioxide in the blood. To accurately measure the blood gases, the physician samples blood directly from an artery. This sampling must be done in this way because only blood that has circulated through the lungs can tell the true oxygen content.

booster: A single shot of a vaccine designed to reawaken the protective response following original immunization.

breath sounds: Sounds heard through a stethoscope; the intensity of the sound of air moving in and out of the lungs indicates the amount of obstruction.

bronchial hygiene: A method to rid the lungs and airways of irritants and retained secretions. It is the act of inhaling a bronchodilator, inhaling moisture when appropriate, and, finally, making expulsive coughing efforts to clear the airway with or without postural drainage maneuvers to facilitate the drainage of secretions.

bronchodilator therapy: The use of drugs that combat musculature spasm of the conducting airways and help to enlarge the constricted airways.

bronchospasm: A sudden narrowing of the airways due in part to contraction of the circular musculature of the conducting airways, in part to inflammatory swelling of the airway lining, and in part to secretions in the airways.

bronchus: The two main divisions of the trachea, one for each lung. These in turn branch some 20 times before the gas exchange membrane is reached. (See Figure 1, Chapter 1.)

capillaries: The smallest blood vessels, which also provide for the exchange of oxygen and carbon dioxide in the lungs. The small capillary branches join to form large vessels that carry oxygenated blood to the tissues.

cartilage: A rigid yet flexible supporting tissue someway similar in structure to bone but without bone's rigidity.

catarrh: The excessive production of mucus associated with a mild chronic cough. This chronic cough and expectoration probably signify chronic bronchitis.

chronic obstructive pulmonary disease (COPD): Also known as chronic obstructive lung disease or chronic airway obstruction. A broad term encompassing emphysema, chronic bronchitis, and/or chronic asthma. Physicians sometimes like to use this somewhat noncommittal term because elements of all three major diseases may be present in a given patient. Probably, more such nonspecific terms will come into use until scientists settle on specific criteria for the diagnosis of emphysema, chronic bronchitis, and chronic asthma (also called asthmatic bronchitis).

cilia: The hairlike structures that line the airways and beat rhythmically away from the lungs to propel the mucus blanket toward the mouth. The cilia are major cleansing mechanisms of the lungs and, thus, an important defense against commonly inhaled irritants.

cor pulmonale: Strain of the right side of the heart accompanying emphysema and chronic bronchitis.

cortisone drugs: A family of anti-inflammatory steroid compounds, including prednisone and a variety of related drugs.

decongestion: The reduction of swelling of nasal passages by nose drops. These function in a manner somewhat similar to inhaled bronchodilators.

diuretics: A group of drugs that promote the kidney's excretion of salt and water including HydroDiuril® (hydrochlorothiazide), Esidrix® (hydrochlorothiazide), Lasix® (furosemide), and a variety of others. No effective diuretic is presently sold over the counter.

dyspnea: The medical term referring to shortness of breath. Literally, dyspnea means "bad breath;" physicians and patients agree that it is bad when you can't get your breath.

edema: Swelling of the extremities caused by salt and water retention. Some patients recognize edema themselves because of tight shoes and stockings. Squeezing on edematous legs leaves an imprint of the thumb or finger.

effluent: Streaming outward from any system, such as moisture from a nebulizer.

elastic superstructure: Interwoven stretchable fibers that connect to the alveoli and conducting airways and aid in inspiration and expiration.

electrocardiogram (EKG): A tracing of the heart's electrical activity; an important indicator of heart strain and other heart diseases. The EKG records the heart's activity, sensing tiny electrical impulses from the heart. The test utilizes electrodes attached to the arms, legs, and chest.

expectorant: A drug that helps thin and remove secretions. The effectiveness of the various expectorants is open to great debate.

genetic: Refers to heredity; one possible cause of emphysema and perhaps bronchitis in the case of AAT deficiency.

heart failure: The inability of the heart to meet its workload. When the heart is strained, its output of blood is diminished, and the kidneys do not receive sufficient circulation to excrete a normal quantity of salt and water. The term "heart failure" does not imply that the heart is hopelessly damaged, but that it is temporarily not doing enough work. Heart failure can be treated with drugs to stimulate the heart (digitalis derivatives). Even more importantly, treatment of a lung condition will often unburden the heart. Diuretics and other drugs will relieve the burden if excessive fluid is present in the body (see edema).

humidification: The act of moisturizing the air with molecules of water.

inflammation: The process of irritation, reddening, and swelling of tissues.

inspiration: The taking of air into the lungs; inhalation.

irritant: Any noxious substance that may damage the lungs.

lymph glands: Pea-sized glands containing lymphatic cells. These glands are an important defense against infection and are also the stations in which irritants like tar are deposited by scavenger cells (macrophages).

lymphatic channels: Delicate vessels that carry the flow of a clear fluid (lymph) to the lymph glands.

macrophage: The scavenger cells of the lung that have the ability to consume and carry away lung irritants.

medulla: The most primitive portion of the brain that contains the centers of vital organ functions, such as the respiratory center in the base of the brain (brain stem).

metabolism: The consumption of oxygen and nutrients for energy production and for the maintenance of body tissues.

mucolytic agent: The term "lytic" refers to an ability to dissolve something. Thus, "mucolytic" implies that we have drugs that can dissolve mucus. This is partly true, but we still do not have the ideal drug to thin secretions.

mucous glands: The glands that normally provide mucus for the cleansing of the lungs. These glands are enlarged in chronic bronchitis. See Organidin®.

nebulizer: A device that breaks liquid into tiny droplets of suitable size for inhalation into the lungs.

oxygen transport: The delivery of oxygen to the tissues; a function of circulation. The term implies normal oxygenation of the blood and the delivery of this oxygenated blood to all the tissues of the body.

panacea: A term referring to a "cure-all." Unfortunately, a panacea does not exist.

particle size: Refers to the size of the nebulized droplets of moisture or of a bronchodilator. Large particles deposit on the larger airways and smaller particles deposit on the narrower airways of the lungs.

pedometer: A device that measures distance in walking. Its appearance is similar to that of a watch; it functions by pendulum to record distance travelled.

phlebotomy: The therapeutic withdrawal of blood; usually a pint is removed, sometimes at intervals.

physiological: Referring to normal body function.

pleura: The thin delicate membrane that encases the lungs and lines the chest cavity.

pneumonia: A sudden infection of localized areas of the lungs; episodes of pneumonia frequently accompany bronchitis.

postural drainage: The act of positioning oneself in certain postures to allow gravity to help drain the lungs.

prophylactic treatment: The term "prophylaxis" refers to prevention; prophylactic antibiotic treatment implies the possibility of preventing infection.

protuberant: Pouching outward, as in allowing the abdomen to pouch outward during inspiration.

red blood cells: The cells that give the blood its red color; they contain hemoglobin and carry oxygen to the tissues.

resistance: In the context of this book, impediments to airflow in and out of the lungs.

respirable-size particles: The smaller particles that can be inhaled and deposited deep into the lungs.

respiration: The act of taking air into the lungs; the delivery of oxygen to the tissues and return of carbon dioxide to the lungs for removal.

respiratory center: An area of the brain that controls respiration; the respiratory center is stimulated by oxygen deficiency and carbon dioxide build-up, as well as by muscular activity.

respiratory failure: The sudden situation in which the lungs are not providing normal oxygenation or normal carbon dioxide removal.

sedative: A drug designed to promote sleep. These drugs are potentially dangerous to patients with chronic lung disease.

side effects: Undesirable reactions to drugs. In the case of steroid drugs, one finds a swelling of the face, salt and water retention, irritation of the stomach occasionally leading to ulcers, and a variety of less common but severe reactions.

somnolence: Excessive sleepiness. May occur from drugs or from severe states of respiratory failure during which the lungs are not providing adequate oxygenation and carbon dioxide removal.

spirometer: A machine that measures breathing capacity. This may be a simple hand-held device that roughly estimates breathing capacity, or it may be a more complicated instrument that appears similar to a tin can that travels up and down with each breath. More elaborate devices are interfaced with computers. (See Chapter 3.)

sputum: Expectorated mucus or phlegm.

stethoscope: The ear piece that physicians use to examine the heart and lungs.

surfactant: A surface-tension material on the alveoli which allows them to open easily, i.e., with little pressure.

tenacious: A term referring to thick, stringy, and difficult-to-remove secretions.

thorax: The muscular and bony structure of the chest.

toxicity: An undesirable result of drug use.

trachea: The main airway (windpipe) supplying both lungs.

tracheostomy: The surgical opening in the main airway, the trachea.

tracheostomy tube: The plastic, rubber, or metal tube placed into the windpipe through a surgical opening.

tranquilizer: A sedative-like drug that is commonly used to reduce anxiety, e.g. Valium (diazepam), Librium (chlordiazepoxide).

vaccine: An injection that may stimulate the immune response to protect an individual from a natural infection.

ventilator: The proper term for a breathing machine used to treat respiratory failure.

virus: A group of highly contagious infectious agents that cause a variety of head colds and chest infections. Viruses are not killed by antibiotics, and thus we usually have no way of preventing or stopping viral infections. Vaccination against the influenza virus, however, is effective.

wheeze: The whistling sound of air entering or leaving the lungs. A sign of muscular spasm of the airways, and a sign of asthma.

white blood cells: The cells that generally combat infection; the white cell count is usually increased with infection.

Index

Page numbers in *italics* refer to illustrations; numbers followed by *t* indicate tables.

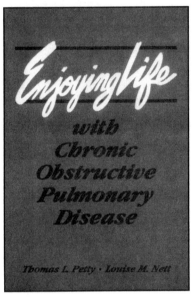

Want Extra Copies of *Enjoying Life With Chronic Obstructive Pulmonary Disease* for your friends or relatives?

If you would like additional copies of this book, or if one of your friends or relatives wants to obtain a copy, they are available at $12.95 each. Make your check or money order payable to Laennec Publishing and mail it to the address below. (Residents of New Jersey, Add 6% sales tax.)

Orders of $38.85 or more (3 or more copies) may be charged on your Mastercard or Visa. Please include your name, account number, expiration date, and indicate Mastercard or Visa.

LAENNEC PUBLISHING, INC.

218 Little Falls Road

Cedar Grove, New Jersey 07009-1231